Marketing
by Objectives
for Hospitals

Robin E. Scott MacStravic, Ph.D.

AN ASPEN PUBLICATION®
Aspen Systems Corporation
Germantown, Maryland
London, England
1980

Library of Congress Cataloging in Publication Data

MacStravic, Robin E.
Marketing by objectives for hospitals.

Includes bibliographies and index.
1. Hospitals—Marketing. I. Title. [DNLM: 1.
Economic, Hospital. 2. Marketing of health
services. WX157 M175m]
RA965.5.M32   362.1'1'0688   80-10903
ISBN 0-89443-174-9

Library of Congress Catalog Card Number: 80-10903
ISBN: 0-89443-174-9

Printed in the United States of America

1 2 3 4 5

Table of Contents

Preface

This book is intended to pick up where its predecessor, *Marketing Health Care,* left off. Where the first book was general and introductory in scope and focus, this one is meant to supply specific conceptual and operational tools that managers and planners can use in implementing marketing efforts in the health field. Specific examples of successful and unsuccessful attempts to manage a health organization's affairs with and without marketing are provided to illustrate the strengths and limitations of current developmental efforts.

It is understandable that most readers will look to marketing as a source of techniques to use in assuring the success of current programs and in promoting successful new ventures. While marketing analysis often may reveal that eliminating or cutting back a program is truly the best choice, the emphasis on new program development and growth is natural and appropriate for a marketing text.

This work is intended to enable its readers to approach developmental opportunities from a realistic and pragmatic perspective. To do so requires a thorough awareness of present and foreseeable realities within the organization and in its environment. The first part of the book is devoted to discussion of what a marketing information base contains and how to develop it. The second part covers the use of marketing concepts and techniques in systematically thinking through the creation of a marketing plan. The third part focuses on the use of marketing in making critical management decisions about the organization's role, resources, and development of a permanent marketing function. The last part offers case examples in which managers of health organizations either did or did not employ marketing in planning and managing their development. It is intended as a representative, though not comprehensive, sampling of how marketing can and will affect the success of health program development.

Many of the ills of the current health system have been traced either to greedy providers or to careless financers of health care. In many ways, however, it has been a failure of the market to select out the best providers and eliminate marginal programs. The combination of health insurance, which significantly reduces consumer choice based on cost, and cost-based reimbursement, which significantly insulates providers from expenditure risk, has enabled the system to get by without marketing. In the future, effective marketing—the careful selection of what to offer and to whom, as well as the successful design and implementation of optimal program features—will dictate who survives and who doesn't. It is hoped that this book will assist the implementation of effective marketing programs.

Robin E. Scott MacStravic
Mercer Island, Washington
April 1980

Acknowledgments

This book owes somewhat less to other writers in the general field of marketing and more to the many authors who have added to the literature on marketing health care in recent years. The author also acknowledges the assistance provided by a number of students in marketing seminars at the University of Washington whose contributions have been very helpful in preparing case materials. A special debt is owed to Bill Bush, whose contributions on promotional strategies are reflected in both the chapter on that subject and its corresponding case. Particular thanks are offered to Cheryl Michels for many of the finishing touches, and to Suellen MacStravic, whose patient and diligent typing helped translate the idea for the book into this reality.

Part I

Information Collection and Analysis

In this part, the design and implementation of information collection and analysis are the focus of discussion. If it can be said that the market functions on money, and the army travels on its stomach, then marketing runs on information. While intuition and informal intelligence processes are useful and no doubt will be used in the majority of situations, a more systematic approach is described here to guide intuition and assist more complex endeavors.

The importance of information to marketing can hardly be overestimated. By definition, marketing requires the understanding of behavior in order to facilitate predicting and influencing such behavior. Unless that understanding is truly intuitive, or unless you're willing to bet on chance alone, a systematic approach to understanding human and organizational motivation is recommended. The approach described in the first four chapters can be used for specific market research efforts geared to specific market decisions, or to initial and incremental attempts at a general marketing data base.

Chapter 1 describes the general idea of the market audit, a comprehensive, systematic format and process for identifying information requirements and evaluating the results. It focuses on five areas: human and organizational behavior, external and internal impacts, psychographic and demographic factors, environmental developments, and the competition. It examines past, present, and future as they involve your relations with important markets: current and prospective patients, actual and prospective medical staff, referring physicians or agencies.

Chapter 2 discusses market research in general, covering how you specify what you want to know, collect data about it, and analyze the results so as to come up with optimal market decisions. It includes descriptions of basic rules and guidelines of research, including population identification, sampling, data collection, and analysis. However, it is designed to make the reader an informed manager and consumer of market research efforts, rather than a researcher.

Chapter 3 identifies and describes the kinds of results you get through a market audit or market research efforts. These include, first, the identification of problems: market relations, causes, or impacts that should be changed lest the health of the organization and its community be damaged. Second are threats: the prospect of potential changes in market relations whose effects would be deleterious to organization or community. Third are opportunities: possible changes the organization might pursue to the expected advantage of organization and community. All are discussed in relation to what to do about them as well as how to recognize them.

Chapter 4 recommends specific procedures for designing and executing market audits or research. It covers a recommended sequence of data collection and analysis from inside the organization to outside, from general to specific, and from a present to a future focus. While it suggests an incremental approach rather than full steam ahead, the timing and scope of each step is up to each organization.

Chapter 1

The Market Audit

An important maxim regarding the use of the marketing in health care planning and development is the paraphrase: "Don't just do something, stand there!" Marketing assumes that data and analysis generally are preferable to intuition or automatic response. It focuses on how and why people and organizations behave in the present and asks whether changes in behavior are likely, desirable, and achievable in the future. It analyzes problems, chooses interventions, and evaluates results. All this requires information.

The first step in gathering the information—the intelligence—to serve as a basis for a marketing effort is the market audit. Usually referred to as a market*ing* audit in most industries, it is essentially a data base to guide marketing decisions. Its fundamental purpose is to examine systematically how well the organization is doing in its market relations. How well things are going in your market includes both a still picture of what things are like right now and a preview of where they seem to be headed in the future.

Both the present and foreseeable future of your market relations are important. The first lets you know whether you have immediate problems or success, the second identifies possible future problems or self-correcting situations that don't require your intervention. A market audit should enable you to identify where your intervention is required and where it will do the most good. It precedes but leads directly to action, toward achieving a desired change or preventing one you'd rather avoid.

AUDIT CONTENT

The market audit contains three major categories of information, each of which has two parts. The major categories are:

1. Behavior: how you behave with respect to your markets and how your markets behave with respect to you. The behavior of specific segments

3

of the market and of your individual programs toward the populations they serve are included in this category. In recognizing the focus of marketing on transactions and on exchange behavior, it is necessary that both parties' behavior be examined.

2. Impact: what happens to your organization because of those two kinds of behavior and what happens to your markets because of their relations, or lack of them, with you. Your impacts may be measured in traditional performance terms while theirs may be reflected in health status measures.

3. Causal factors: these include both demographic and psychographic characteristics of your markets that may aid you in predicting, evaluating, or influencing their behavior. You may use such characteristics to identify separable market segments and to forecast their probability of demanding specific services or of preferring one of alternative sources of that service.

In addition to these three internal market factors, two external items are worth mentioning. First is the environment—elements likely to be beyond your direct control that affect the behavior of your markets. Environmental factors may include developments in the economy, in regulatory efforts, governmental policy (e.g., national health insurance), medical technology, or other areas likely to alter how your markets relate to you. The other external factor is your competition—any organization that offers roughly similar benefits to potentially the same markets you now serve or hope to serve. You should view your competition broadly, not restricting consideration to similar organizations, but including all organizations or individual providers that are in roughly the same business.

Examples of competitors in the primary medical care business include:

- hospitals: emergency rooms, outpatient departments, primary care centers
- neighborhood health centers
- public health clinics
- health maintenance organizations
- private practitioners
- industrial clinics

The behavior of your competition toward your current and potential markets, and of your markets toward your competitors, is an important audit component.

IMPACT

While behavior is the focus of marketing efforts, the organization probably will wish to begin designing its audit with impacts. This is a reasonable approach and helps the organization focus its thinking. The starting point for determining what kind of impacts to look at, what performance characteristics to audit, in most cases will be the organization's mission, role, and program. If the mission statement, goals, and objectives are vague and global (e.g., serve the health needs of the community), it will take some work to translate them into performance measures. Where they are more precise (e.g., maintain 80 percent occupancy, break even on all programs), the job is much simpler.

The two classes of impacts—what determines how successful an organization is—are the effects the organization has on its publics and the effects its publics have on the organization. In the first category are such factors as:

- the health of the community or particular market segments such as indigent vs. affluent, ethnic groups, mothers and children, residents of a particular area, etc.; these measures reflect the organization's purpose and target communities.
- the satisfaction of such communities with the services provided by the organization
- the reputation of the organization in the wider community, its level of acceptance and support by people other than current patients or clients; the attitudes of specific segments such as potential donors, political figures, regulatory agencies, etc., may be of special interest

It must be recognized that such success or performance impact measures also have *causal* importance. Your organization's reputation clearly can have some influence on how people behave toward you. The satisfaction of your patients will influence their behavior toward you and your reputation. Your impact on health will influence both satisfaction and reputation. The designation of these factors as impact measures does not ignore these complex realities, it merely provides a starting point for identifying such measures.

Specific measures for your impact on health may include vital statistics on the population you serve (mortality and morbidity data) and your own measures of quality (surgical mortality or complications rates, incidence of preventable diseases, etc.). If your organization justifies its existence in terms of protecting or improving the health of some specific set of persons, it should be monitoring some measures of health to keep track of how well you're doing. These should include both positive impact measures (declining infant mortality, reductions in disease-specific mortality) and negative impact measures (iatrogenic conditions, nosocomial infections).

Measures of your reputation in the community or your patients' satisfaction with your programs will require you to collect original data. Specific techniques and considerations in market research are discussed in Chapter 2. Basically, your audit should ask what people know about you and how they feel about you as the result of your general contribution to the community or your specific contribution to individuals and their families.

The second category of impacts in the market audit involves those the patient and general community have upon you. These should include measures that reflect the health of the organization itself: financial factors especially, but also measures of efficiency and internal effectiveness. Traditional examples among financial measures include expenditures, revenues, and their relationship for specific programs as well as overall cash flow, receivables, debt ratios, acid tests, etc. Factors such as occupancy levels, numbers of patients turned away, delayed or rescheduled surgery, etc., will indicate internal effectiveness or efficiency. Such measures result from the interaction of your behavior with your patients' behavior but also may affect your impacts in terms of satisfaction and reputation.

Internal measures for the most part should be available through your own records. Financial data, occupancy levels, productivity figures, and so on should be collected and analyzed routinely. Occasionally, you may wish to devote special efforts to study some aspect of your performance not routinely monitored. Each organization should develop, collect, and examine its own measures of how well its internal operations are going. An example of a specific organization—a hospital corporation—and its market audit effort is discussed in Chapter 13. A sample format is provided at the end of this chapter.

BEHAVIOR

All of your impact measures can and should be understood as the results of some behaviors. Your behavior with respect to patients and the community affects their health status and satisfaction and your reputation and expenditures. Their behavior with respect to you affects your occupancy, revenue, productivity, etc. How you behave with respect to them affects how they behave with respect to you, and vice versa. This is the reality upon which marketing specifically focuses your attention. The identification of which behavior by what people determines your impacts is the crucial challenge and contribution of the market audit.

Who?

The first step in measuring and analyzing behavior is to designate whose behavior interests you. The community and actual patients should be divided into market segments for the purpose of analysis and strategy development. A market segment is simply a set of persons (or organizations):

- who are sufficiently alike to be treated as a homogeneous group and
- who are sufficiently different from others to be treated as a distinct group

The numbers and types of market segments you designate are purely a matter of judgment. The more there are, the more complex your analysis becomes, but the more focused your strategies can be.

Some examples of the kinds of factors that may unite a segment internally and distinguish it from other segments are the following:

Community: Patients

- age (< 15, 15-44, 45-64, 65+, etc.)
- sex (combined with age cohorts)
- race
- residence
- income level
- insurance coverage
- diagnoses
- employment
- religious preference
- marital status
- physician identification

Organization: Employees

- department
- type of employee
- length of service
- union vs. nonunion
- shift
- function/service
- unit

In addition to the community and patient market, you should segment the physician and referral agency markets:

Physician

- location
- specialty
- size of practice
- age
- group vs. solo
- medical staff status
- privileges

Referring Agency

- location
- function/service
- community served
- funding source

The sole purpose of segmenting a population is to treat each segment differently either in your analysis or, later, your market strategy—and preferably both. Distinctions that make no difference are to be avoided. Such classic habits as dividing the community into primary, secondary, and tertiary service areas, if not accompanied by treating each differently in some significant way, are a waste of time and effort. Segmenting should be done not for its own sake but only because and if it aids organizations in understanding, predicting, and influencing the behaviors that concern them.

What?

The *what* of behavior in the market audit should cover all those behaviors that are understood to lead to important impacts. For patients, the behaviors are likely to include:

- admissions rates
- length of stay
- visits per year
- whether they pay bills, what portion they pay, and how long they take to pay

- compliance with regimen or advice
- appointment keeping or breaking, or tardiness

For physicians and referral agencies, the behavior is likely to include:

- patients admitted or referred to you
- total patients admitted or referred anywhere
- length of stay or visits per patient/registrant
- diagnosis mix of admission/referrals
- patient days or visits generated
- revenue generated vs. charges
- expenditures generated vs. costs

Each behavior should be capable of being evaluated in terms of its impact upon the organization's performance. The numbers and types of physicians on a hospital's medical staff and how many of what kinds of patients they refer or admit determine a hospital's census levels, expenditures, and, ultimately, revenue. The amounts and kinds of services provided by your employees determine both expenditures and patient satisfaction. Often a mix of behaviors rather than a single one will affect a given impact but it is that impact that determines how desirable or appropriate the behaviors are. Each behavior monitored or studied should be linked to its single or multiple direct or indirect impacts. Behaviors that cannot be linked to performance impact probably need not be included in the audit.

CAUSAL FACTORS

Just as each behavior should be linked to its impact(s), so, too, should it be linked to potential causal factors. The first set of causal factors may have been partially identified already in the attributes used to determine market segments. Demographic characteristics of markets are useful in two ways:

1. in identifying segments that are distinct from each other and warrant your separate treatment
2. in explaining or predicting how different individuals or organizations behave

Demographic characteristics of patients should be useful in understanding or predicting their disease or injury patterns, what use of health services they make, how much they can or will pay for specific services, and where they will look for such services. Demographic characteristics of physicians or referral agencies should be useful in understanding or predicting how many patients they will admit or refer, of what types, how many services they will prescribe for those patients, and where they will tend to send them. Anticipating future changes in such demographic factors can help your organization predict future changes in behavior and respond to them.

Patients' demographic factors include age, sex, race, education, income, insurance coverage, religious preference, place of residence, and employment. Much of these data are available from your records on actual patients or census data for potential patients. Demographic attributes of physicians that might interest you include age, sex, race, specialty, medical school, internship and residency training, specialty board status, type of practice (single, specialty, or multispecialty group, partnership or solo) office location, and residence. Such data should be available from your records on physicians on your medical staff, from state licensing boards, or from the American Medical Association.

Such demographic factors may help you understand and predict behavior by patients and physicians, but not completely. Psychographic factors—what people know or believe and how they feel about things—also are important. Moreover, while demographic factors can be predicted and responded to, psychographic factors can be targeted specifically for change. You can change what people know and believe about you by supplying information or improving communications. You can change how people feel about you by changing how you behave toward them. Specific approaches to achieving such changes are discussed in Chapter 7, with examples in Chapter 16.

Psychographic factors include what people know and believe about health:

- symptom recognition
- awareness of medical responses
- recognition of "emergencies"
- usefulness of immunization
- risks and hazards in the environment
- risks and hazards in their own behavior

They also include what individuals know and believe about you. Such knowledge and beliefs will fall into one of three categories that are important to your marketing strategy: product, place, and price. *Product* is defined as the benefits people believe they will derive out of doing business with you, being your patient, or becoming a member of your medical staff, for example. *Place* includes the understanding people have about how to go about doing business with you and the circumstances under which they can avail themselves of your product. *Price* is the flip side of product: the financial, physical, and psychological costs to people of doing business with you.

Product factors:

- what services you offer to people
- what good they will do them
- what quality of care you provide
- how modern and complete is your equipment
- how modern, spacious, and clean is your facility
- how qualified and courteous is your staff
- whether staff members care about your patients as people

Note: For physicians you may try to recruit, such factors include both the benefits you offer their patients and the benefits you offer to physicians:

- surgical facility, equipment, and staff
- operating room schedules
- privileges
- perquisites such as physician lounges, dinners for spouses, guarantees of income, etc.
- prospects of responsible positions on the medical staff
- prospects of financial success in the community

Place factors

- hours and days of service availability
- types of people (or physicians) eligible
- types of people (or physicians) welcomed
- convenience of location
- availability of parking
- waiting time for appointments
- waiting time to be seen
- length of time to process application

Price factors:

- out-of-pocket charges/costs to patients
- length of time allowed for payment
- pain or discomfort involved in your services
- personal indignities or psychological discomforts involved
- committee assignments and scutwork required of physicians

As psychographic factors, it matters not so much whether individuals' "knowledge" and beliefs are true but whether they perceive them to be true. The purpose of auditing psychographic factors among your actual or potential customers is to find out what they believe to be true about you. If they are correct in their beliefs and their behavior is affected adversely, you will have to change how you behave. If they are incorrect, but behave accordingly, you may be able to change their beliefs through communication of information. Clearly, it is worth knowing what people perceive and how it affects their behavior in evaluating your current market situation or alternative marketing strategies.

In addition to individuals' knowledge and beliefs about you, psychographic factors include their feelings or attitudes and how they value different product, place, and price factors. In attempting to understand behavior, you want to know why people prefer one behavior over another, choose one source of care over another. Marketing theory holds that most, if not all, behavior can be understood in terms of an exchange. People act so as to get the most they can for what they have to give up in return. To know what is most and what they give up, you must be able to appreciate product, place, and price from their perspective.

Specific approaches to discovering how people feel about you or health or things in general are discussed in Chapter 2. The kinds of feelings you'd be interested in knowing about are likely to include:

- how people rank in importance such factors as convenience, quality, caring, and cost in deciding whether and where to seek services
- how they feel about your organization and its "image"
- what they'd like you to change about yourself
- how they think they'd behave if you did make changes
- how they feel about other organizations offering similar benefits (your competition)

Psychographic information, in contrast to demographic, seldom is likely to be available from records or other secondary sources. To find out what people believe and how they feel, you must anticipate collecting original information. Therefore, you must be selective and pragmatic about how much information you attempt to collect about how many segments of the patient or physician population. Specific guidance for making such decisions is offered in Chapter 2. It must be remembered, however, that while more information may be desirable before making any decision, some decisions have to be made now. Information has costs as well as benefits, and judgment is necessary in realizing that it's time to decide and that more information won't help that much.

The list of items to be included in a market audit is potentially endless, since more information regarding more things about more people is almost always of some value. The most important thing to remember about the audit, however much data you collect, is to be sure you can relate items of information to each other. Specifically, you will want to link demographic and psychographic information to one another to know exactly who believes and feels how. You will wish to link causal factors to specific behaviors: to understand how your behavior affects their attitudes and subsequent behavior and to understand and predict how different people (demographics) with different knowledge, beliefs, and attitudes are likely to behave in the future. You most certainly will need to know how specific behaviors affect your performance.

The interactions among these components of market audit are displayed graphically in Figure 1-1 (arrows portray flow and direction of interactions). For example, your treatment of patients (behavior) may affect how they feel about you (psychographics) and whether they return for care (behavior) and receive maximum benefit (impact on them). It also may affect whether they pay their bills or sue you for malpractice (behavior) and what that does to you financially (impact on you). A market audit not only must ascertain the facts about causes, behavior, and impacts, but also must produce analyses that clarify how they affect each other.

Data on the demographic and psychographic characteristics of a patient or physician population that can't be linked to differences in behavior are virtually worthless. Data on different behaviors, by you and by them, that can't be

---

Figure 1-1 Interactions Among Market Audit Elements

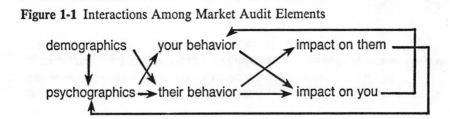

linked back to psychographic differences and forward to performance and impact differences, are interesting but of limited decision-making value. It would be better to have fewer data, thoroughly interrelated, than more that are hopelessly isolated.

EXTERNALITIES

In addition to the data you gather and analyze on your current market relations, two other categories of information are necessary in the market audit. First is the analysis of the environment, identifying what is happening out there that will affect how you and your markets interact in the future. Second is analysis of the competition, determining how it now interacts with its markets and what kinds of changes in its market relations are foreseeable or probable in the future.

Environment

Environmental factors include all developments external to the specific people and organizations with which you interact that might alter that interaction in the future. They cover such direct and obvious developments as governmental regulation, planning and rate-setting agencies, educational institutions, licensing agencies, national health insurance, developments in the overall economy, changes in medical technology, or trends in health. Any such developments that might alter your behavior or that of your markets significantly should be assessed, as should the market-specific demographic and psychographic factors already discussed.

Identifying such factors and forecasting future developments has to be done carefully, since forecasting involves unavoidable uncertainty. Group processes may be useful in identifying important developments, evaluating the probability of their occurrence, and predicting their overall impact on your market relations. Suggestions for forecasting are discussed in detail in Chapter 4. The important point to remember is to focus forecasting on the specific effects you anticipate on your market relations: how you behave with respect to your markets and how they behave with respect to you.

Competition

Other organizations that currently or potentially offer similar benefits (products) to similar markets also should be included in your market audit. Ideally, you would like to have a copy of their audits, telling you how they and their markets behave, what impacts such behaviors have, and what factors explain why customers choose them over you. Some of this information you can get from published data such as their annual reports, the American Hospital Association's Guide issue, and public records on data that must be furnished to governmental agencies and made available to the public. In some cases, such organizations' plans may be published, though probably with the intention of scaring you off rather than providing you with market intelligence about them.

In addition to public records, you may learn of your competitors' market relations through informal, even casual, conversations with them or through persons who have market relationships with both you and them. Physicians who are on the medical staff of more than one hospital or refer to colleagues at other institutions may be informed about what's going on there. Patients who use your services as well as theirs may describe their experiences there. Members of your governing or advisory boards may have some knowledge of what competing organizations are doing or planning.

A more formal source of information on your competitors' market relations would be a survey of the general community. By dividing responses from a community survey into persons who use the competition vs. those who use your services, you can get an idea of how the two groups behave, how they differ, and how well you're doing relative to the competition. No effective marketing program can be carried out in isolation. Whatever you propose doing has to be examined in relation to what the competition is doing or might do (see Chapter 9).

AUDIT RESULTS

The output of the market audit should be a thorough and accurate description of how specific groups of persons behave, what characteristics might explain that behavior, and what impact this has upon the groups themselves and upon your organization. It should tell you what kinds of activities you're doing well, both in terms of their impact and in terms of how your behavior is perceived by others. It also should tell you what you're not doing so well and where you might wish to focus attention. It should help you understand why your performance—your contribution to the community and to the health of your organization—is good, bad, or indifferent.

To evaluate the data output of the market audit, it is necessary to judge, not simply collect, information. You may evaluate the facts you develop by comparing them to specific standards. You probably will have fairly precise expectations for impacts such as the health status of your target community and its satisfaction levels. Similarly, precise standards are likely for internal performance factors such as financial outcomes, occupancy, and total service.

You also may have predetermined expectations for behavior, both yours and theirs, such as seeing every emergency room patient within one minute of arrival for triage, or attracting 80 percent of your target community as registrants.

Even in the absence of specific standards or expectations, you should judge the realities you discover on some basis. A formal or informal group process may be used to examine the results of the audit and decide what's good, bad, and indifferent. If the linkages between causal factors, behavior, and impacts are sufficiently well-established, you should be able to judge demographic and psychographic factors in terms of how they affect behavior and how that behavior results in desirable or undesirable impacts.

The usefulness and application of market audit results are discussed in Chapter 3. Basically, the audit when first conducted should tell you what present and foreseeable realities can be left alone and which ones require your attention. When repeated periodically, the audit will enable you to monitor the effects of your overall or target-specific marketing strategies, and tell you which ones are working how well.

It may take some time to design, convince everyone of the usefulness of, implement, and analyze the kind of market audit that will be most valuable to you and your organization. Your earliest attention ought to be given to the audit, however, as the essential data base for all your marketing efforts. Examples of what can happen should you act without such a data base are given in Chapters 15 and 18. Discussions of how a market audit could have enhanced present and future performance in even successful marketing efforts are provided in Chapters 14 and 16. Specific examples of early and subsequent designs and output of a hospital market audit are presented in Chapter 13.

SUMMARY

The market audit is the first essential step in an effective marketing program. It is designed to tell you how things are going both at present and in the foreseeable future as a basis for your deciding whether and where to intervene. It includes three major categories of information, each of which has two parts: (1) behavior: yours toward your markets and theirs toward you; (2) impact of that behavior: yours and theirs, on them and you; (3) causal factors: demographic and psychographic characteristics that help you understand, predict, and influence behavior.

Impact measures frequently are the starting place for a market audit since they cover situations whose importance to you is clear and about which you most likely have substantial information. They include whatever tells you whether you're having the desired impacts on the community: its health status, satisfaction, and whatever is called for by your mission, role, purpose, goals, and objectives. They also include how healthy your organization is: its output of services, financial health, and community support. You should audit both impacts you are pleased with (e.g., positive health effects) and results you'd not be pleased to find (e.g., negative health effects). To understand such impacts fully, you must be able to relate them to behavior—yours and theirs.

Behavioral factors cover all aspects of how you and your markets behave that have significant links to the impacts about which you're concerned. If your markets' behavior impacts on their own health (e.g., smoking, drinking, driving, exercise, nutrition) and you are concerned with their health, you monitor such behavior. If it impacts on your health (admissions, registrations, payment of bills), you monitor that, too. If your behavior affects their health (surgical mortality or complications, incidence of preventable disease) or if it affects your health (unused capacity, expenditures), you keep track of yours as well. If your behavior affects how your markets behave (you make them wait too long, they stop coming), you care about that.

Causal factors include demographic attributes that help you understand, predict, and influence such behavior. Any factors that are linked significantly to differences in behavior or can be modified to alter current or potential behavior substantially should be included in the audit. While demographic information should be available from your own or public records, psychographic data will require significant original effort.

Besides data on your markets and your specific interactions with them, the market audit examines two external factors: the overall environment and the competition. Through identifying general trends and developments that will affect future market relations, you can predict and prepare for changes in such relations. Through identifying how your competition and its market relations are going plus what plans it has, you can determine most effectively where you can succeed in terms of viable markets and services. No market audit is complete without these two important externalities.

The result of a market audit should be a thorough, clear picture of your current and foreseeable relations with your markets. It should be useful to you in identifying where your intervention is unnecessary, potentially useful, or absolutely required. The audit, when repeated, will enable you to monitor the results of your interventions and to prepare responses in advance of crises. To obtain full benefit of the audit, it is essential that each of the components be linked to the others, so you can understand how they interact. Only by understanding the dynamics of causes, behavior, and impacts in all directions can you make the most effective use of audit information.

SUGGESTIONS FOR MARKET AUDIT

Step 1. Identify the specific set of market transactions you want to audit—e.g., inpatient utilization by service.

Step 2. Identify the specific behaviors you're interested in measuring:
  A. Patients

	Current	Past Years

    admissions
    length of stay
    average daily census (ADC)
    variability of census (standard deviation)
    ancillary service use
  B. Physicians
    number of admissions
    length of stay
    vacation timing
    ancillary service use
    numbers of physicians on staff

Step 3. Describe how you behave with respect to this market:
  A. Patients
    number of people wait-listed
    average length of wait for admission
    number of patients placed in "wrong" units
    proportion of time unit was understaffed/overstaffed
    percent of meals served hot, on time, etc.
  B. Physicians
    admitting privilege rules
    priorities
    perquisites
    percent of admissions delayed
    percent of surgeries cancelled
    emergency room coverage required
    committee responsibilities

Step 4. Evaluate current behavior and current direction of change in terms of hospital performance/success measures:
    occupancy rate
    lost patient days because of lack of beds
    total revenue this service

total expenses this service
total estimated lost revenue due to lost patients, if any
revenue contributions to other services
expenditure contributions to other services
payments as percent of charges
receivables rate

Step 5. Identify patients' demographic and psychographic factors of interest that might explain behavior or be focused on to change it.

Demographic: age, sex, race, income, health insurance coverage, employment, size of family, residence, family physician, religious preference

Psychographic: knowledge of hospital's services, attitudes toward quality, cost, personal aspects of care received, understanding of condition, feelings about doctors, nurses, hospital

---

Readings

Market Audit in Health

Ewell, C. "Practical Plagiarism for Health Services Administration," *American Journal of Public Health* 64:3, March 1974, p. 233.

Ewing, R. "Getting Back in Touch with the Community: A Task for Trustees." *Trustee* 30:11, November 1977, p. 36.

Kotler, P. "From Sales Obsession to Marketing Effectiveness." *Harvard Business Review*, November/December 1977, p. 67.

Lovelock, C. "Concepts and Strategies for Health Marketers." *Hospital and Health Services Administration* 22:4, Fall 1977, p. 50.

MacStravic, R. "The Health Care Market Audit." *Hospital Progress*, October 1978.

Audit in Other Industries

Alderson, W., and Green, P. *Planning and Problem-Solving in Marketing.* Homewood, Ill.: Richard D. Irvin, 1964, p. 390.

Bauer, R., and Fenn, D. "What Is a Corporate Social Audit?" *Harvard Business Review*, January/February 1973, p. 37.

Gilbert, A.C. "A Victim of Poor Quality, Timing, Product Planning." *Marketing Insights*, March 6, 1967, p. 10.

Kelley, E.J., *Marketing Planning and Competitive Strategy.* Englewood Cliffs, N.J.: Prentice-Hall, Inc., 1972, p. 121.

Kotler, P., and Lopata, R. (Britt, S., ed.) "The Marketing Audit." *Marketing Manager's Handbook,* Chicago: Dartnell Corp., 1973, p. 1074.

Sessions, R. "What a Soundly Conducted Marketing Audit Can Accomplish." *Analyzing and Improving Marketing Performance,* Report No. 32. New York: American Management Association, 1959, p. 20.

Smith, R. "Standards for Appraisal for the Marketing Audit." Ibid., p. 48.

Suchmer, A. "The Marketing Audit, Its Nature, Purposes and Problems." Ibid., p. 13.

Impacts

Fryzel, R. "Marketing Nonprofit Institutions." *Hospital and Health Services Administration* 23:1, Winter 1978, p. 8.

Hogan, S. "Your Patient Mix Affects Costs." *Hospital Financial Management,* April 1978, p. 20.

"Operational Auditing Can Help Hospital Evaluate Effectiveness, Efficiency and Economy." *Hospitals, JAHA* 52, March 1, 1978, p. 46.

Ross, D., and Tripoli, F. "Fiscal Risks, Methods, Rewards Shape Community Outreach Success." *Hospitals, JAHA* 51, July 16, 1977, p. 86.

Behavior

Karr, D. "Increasing a Hospital's Market Share." *Hospitals, JAHA* 51, June 1, 1971, p. 64.

Roberts, S. "Improving Primary Care Clinic's Effectiveness Through Assessment." *Hospitals, JAHA* 51, Nov. 1, 1977, p. 123.

Zimmerman, J. "Service Areas and Their Needs Must Be Reassessed." *Hospitals, JAHA* 49, September 1, 1975, p. 46.

Zuckerman, A. "Patient Origin Study Profiles Service Area, Evolving Patterns." *Hospitals, JAHA,* July 16, 1977, p. 83.

Causes

Flexner, W., et al. "Discovering What the Health Consumer Really Wants." *Health Care Management Review* 2:4, Fall, 1977, p. 43.

Koutsopoulos, K., et al. "Psychometric Modeling of Consumer Decisions in Primary Health Care." *Health Services Research* 12:4, Winter, 1977, p. 427.

Stratmann, W. "A Study of Consumer Attitudes About Health Care." *Medical Care* 13:7, July 1975, p. 537.

Tanaka, A. "Problems Facing Rural Physicians." *Federation Bulletin* 65:1, January 1978, p. 3.

Externalities

Creditor, M. and U. "The Ecology of an Urban Voluntary Hospital: The Referral Chain." *Medical Care* 10:1, January/February 1972, p. 88.

Cunningham, R. "Face Fewer Admissions, Shorter Stays." *Modern Healthcare,* June 1977, p. 29.

Ranieri, W. "Cross-Cutting Health Priorities: A Management Trap." *Hospital and Health Services Administration* 22:4, Fall 1977, p. 24.

Seaver, D. "Hospital Reverses Role, Reaches Out to Cultivate and Capture Markets." *Hospitals, JAHA,* June 1, 1977, p. 59.

Chapter 2

Market Research

To carry out the market audit or to discover important facts about your current and potential markets at any time, the ability to perform market research is essential. Market research is simply research into markets. It contains few unique requirements or methods not part of conventional survey research. However, some analytical techniques that are specific to market research are described in this chapter. The focus of market research is on understanding behavior, its causes, and its impacts, so it is essential to the market audit.

The behavior of greatest interest in market research is that of consumers, although any group whose behavior toward your organization is worth understanding can be the focus. Certainly, understanding the motivations and behavior of physicians and referral, planning, and regulatory agencies would be worthwhile. It is entirely possible for market research to be used to understand the behavior of current and potential employees, volunteers, or board members as well.

The appropriate sequence in the design of market research is to:

1. identify a decision or set of decisions you plan to make
2. determine what facts, projections, or feelings it would be useful for you to know about in making that decision
3. decide what analyses, comparisons, and formulas would give you the best estimates of the facts, projections, and feelings you want to know
4. identify what specific pieces of data are required to perform the analysis
5. determine what population, sample, data collection, and scaling technique will produce the pieces of data required for analysis

1. DECISION

The purpose of any data collection effort is to help you make a decision. By specifying precisely what the decision is, you can design your research most appropriately to help you make the most informed choice. The market audit is a nonspecific research effort, lacking any precise decision focus. For this reason, the facts, projections, and feelings are more difficult to describe than if some decision were in mind. In other cases where market research is to be carried out, however, the instigation is likely to come from the necessity of making a decision. The results of the audit itself may well suggest the desirability of some choice of action, requiring further, more intensive study.

The decision should be an action one, related to developing, expanding, reducing, or eliminating some service, approaching a new market, or embarking on a public relations effort. In effect, the process involves asking yourself: before I decide what to do, what do I want to know? It is having in mind some action that prompts your asking questions and should direct you as to which questions to ask.

2. FACTS, FORECASTS, FEELINGS

In examining a prospective decision, a choice among alternative actions, or simply whether or not to act, three types of information are of interest to you: facts (demographics, behavior, impacts), feelings (psychographics and some impacts), and forecasts (everything). Decisions are made based on the combination of what the current situation is and would become without your action, and what the situation would become as the result of your intervention. Any marketing situation involves the categories of behavior, impacts, and causal factors, though only the market audit requires a comprehensive examination of all three.

In deciding whether to act about overuse of a hospital emergency room, for example, you would want to know what damage is being done to your organization and its mission (impacts) because of what type and extent of E.R. abuse (behavior). In assessing particular strategies, you might wish to identify exactly who uses the E.R. improperly (demographics) and what prompts them to do so (psychographics). Such external factors as insurance provisions (environmental) or the behavior of local physicians (competition) also should enter into your thinking.

In simplest terms, your market research is aimed at helping you anticipate what will happen to the current situation if you maintain business as usual vs. what will happen if you follow any alternative course of action. The differences between action and inaction, in terms of their costs and benefits to you and your organization's health and mission, will provide the basis for making an action decision. Since forecasting clearly is a part of this analysis, you must deal with the future as well as the present. (See Chapter 4 for specific techniques.)

3. ANALYTICAL OPTIONS

Having decided what facts, forecasts, and feelings you need to know as part of reaching a decision, you then should choose the form of analysis you plan to use in establishing these inputs. Such analysis may be as simple as a comparison between two measures such as ratios or rates or as complex as some multivariate analysis (see Chapter 4). It is important to identify first the form of analysis you intend to use before you determine the specific items of data you wish to collect. The most wasteful approach would be to collect data first, then realize how little of it is appropriate for the proposed analysis.

Both the form of the analysis and its place in your decision should be known at the outset in order to determine how much time and effort should be spent in collecting data. Each analytical form will have its own special data requirements, which means its value would be compromised if less than appropriate data were employed. The use of cross-sectional data (about different places at the same time) to make longitudinal estimates (about the same place at a different time) is a classic and common example of analysis compromised by data.

4. DATA REQUIREMENTS

The data specified for collection should be identified precisely and unambiguously. It should be clear whether you are asking for facts or feelings, in the present or future, about exactly whom. Are you trying to establish who, what, where, when, how, or why? Do you need income data in precise terms or ranges? Are you interested in determining how many persons ever use your services, what percentage of the total community they represent, or how frequently your patients use a given service? Each requires significantly different though related data.

Data requirements must be specified in such a way as to fit precisely into the mode of analysis you intend to use. To obtain rates or ratios, for example, you must make sure that data in the numerator (behavior such as admissions visits) match data in the denominator (the precise population at risk), or that the number of events you counted match the time frame you're using. This may seem a straightforward and obvious requirement but it is one of the most common sources of analytical problems in practice.

An outpatient department that counts visits but not individuals, for example, may greatly overestimate the number of persons it serves and underestimate the rate of visits per person per year. Annual patient days of care can be estimated erroneously from discharge data if some patients stay for extended periods in a long-term care facility.

5. DATA COLLECTION

The remainder of this chapter is devoted to some simple rules of data collection. They represent what persons who may plan and receive the results of research ought to know, rather than what a survey researcher would know. For those who want to learn more about the details of carrying out a data collection effort, some readings are suggested at the end of this chapter. It would be impossible to cover such details in a part of one chapter here, however.

Population

The first requirement in data collection is to identify precisely the population, the set of factors or persons, on which you wish to collect data. Whether this covers inpatients or outpatients, current or prospective patients, all physicians or only active medical staff must be specified initially. A count must be made of this population to determine whether all can or should be measured or examined in terms of a specific data requirement. If the number of persons is sufficiently small, or the importance of getting precise data about each member sufficiently great, all should be included in the data collection effort.

Sample

Sampling is a relatively simple area with well-known quantitative guidelines but one not well understood by most health decisionmakers. When a population is too large to permit examining every member, a sample must be chosen. Both the type of sample and its size are important and subject to fairly rigid rules. The greatest errors in market research occur because of improperly drawn or inadequate-sized samples. The mysterious-sounding but fairly simple rules of sampling theory are worth mastering to prevent misguiding research efforts or being misguided by improper research results.

The essential requirement of sampling is to make certain that the sample used is truly representative of the population about which you're concerned. This involves ensuring two things:

1. that the sample be drawn from the population in a statistically reliable fashion, using simple or stratified random sampling or an equally accepted technique
2. that the sample be of sufficient size to warrant whatever inference you make from it to the population at large

There are many ways in which a sample may be drawn improperly. Interviewing the first 20 persons who come to your agency or program may bias results if early arrivals tend to differ from later ones. Samples of convenience, such as using passers-by or the few who will stop and answer your questions to estimate general public attitudes are to be avoided. The most common examples of improperly drawn samples occur in general mailings of questionnaires. However appropriately you may have selected who will get the questionnaires (e.g., the entire population of interest or random sample), those who respond are self-selected and may differ from those who didn't reply.

If you send out 1,000 questionnaires and get 200 returns, half of whom express one opinion or report some trait, and half of whom don't, you have a number of choices. You can assume that the 800 persons who didn't respond split exactly the same way, and estimate that the population as a whole divides 50-50. You also can assume that every one of the nonrespondents has one opinion, and the only exceptions are the 100 in your respondents who expressed the opposite opinion. This would lead you to conclude that 90 percent of the population thinks one way vs. 10 percent the other.

There are virtually endless possibilities for treating nonrespondents, none of them very good. For convenience's sake you may make almost any assumption you wish about those who didn't reply. The safest assumption is always that they differ in some respect from those who did, or else you would have received either a 0 percent or 100 percent response rate. Any other assumption you make may be erroneous.

In general, it is better to use smaller samples and get nearly 100 percent responses wherever possible, rather than larger samples with low response rates, even if the latter produce more returns. It is not the number of persons or items of information that is important, but how well they represent the entire population in which you're interested. Anything less than 100 percent response from a sample introduces at least the possibility of bias. The greater the proportion of the sample about which you learn nothing, the greater the possibility and potential extent of bias.

Even a small sample can produce accurate estimates of current reality and useful forecasts of future reality. The traditional 1,600-person samples used by the Gallup and Lou Harris polls are a classic example of this. Most of the errors produced by such relatively small samples (in terms of representing more than 200 million people) arise from their use to predict future behavior (voting) rather than estimate current reality.

The size of a sample required to give confident and precise estimates of facts and feelings within a population can be calculated through a relatively simple formula. The reasoning behind this formula is that results taken from different samples of the same population will differ over a narrow and predictable range. If 50 percent of the population at large is male, and 50 percent female, samples of 100 persons selected at random will produce proportions ranging from 40 percent to 60 percent in 19 out of 20 cases (95 percent confidence). Samples of 400 will produce results from 45 percent to 55 percent in 95 percent of the cases.

The formula for determining sample size is based on the fact that larger samples produce greater precision and that the increase in precision is proportional to the square root of the sample size. A sample four times as big gives you twice the precision, or half the range of error.

If you are estimating proportions, what share of the population is, behaves, or thinks one way vs. another, the formula for sample size is as follows:

$$S = \left(\frac{1.96\,d}{e} \right)^2$$

where   S = sample size required
         d = the standard deviation of the proportion
         e = the error you're willing to accept, e.g., ± e

The standard deviation of a proportion is calculated as:

$$\sqrt{p \times (1 - p)}$$

where   p = the proportion (50% = .50)

Mathematically, the highest a standard deviation for a proportion can get is $\sqrt{.25}$. This occurs when the split is even and p = .50. Standard deviation equals $\sqrt{(.5) \times (1 - .5)} = \sqrt{.25}$. If the actual proportion is anything other than .5, the standard deviation is less. If the proportion is .40 for example, the standard deviation is $\sqrt{(.40)\,(.60)} = \sqrt{.24}$. For proportions of .2, standard deviation is $\sqrt{(.2)\,(.8)} = \sqrt{.16}$. As proportions get extremely small, standard deviations get even smaller. For a proportion of .05, the standard deviation would be only $\sqrt{(.05)\,(.95)} = \sqrt{.0475}$.

Thus, the worst case, in terms of sample size requirements, would be where the proportion is .5 or close to it. If you don't have any idea what the proportion really is, therefore, you can use this estimate as the most conservative choice and be sure your sample size will produce results at least as accurate as you wish.

For example, if you want to estimate the proportion of the population that prefers your organization to others, or earns more than \$15,000 per year, or smokes, and you need to be accurate to within ± 5 percent (.05), you would use the formula as follows:

$$S = \left(\frac{2 * d}{e} \right)^2$$

d (estimated) = .50
e (your choice) = .05

$$S = \left(\frac{2 \times .50}{.05} \right)^2$$

$$= \left(\frac{1}{.05} \right)^2$$

$$= 20^2$$
$$= 400$$

Thus you'd need a maximum sample of 400 persons to estimate the proportion of a population that is, acts, or thinks one way vs. another, with an accuracy of ± 5 percent and assurance that you'd be wrong only once in 20 times. In general, where proportions can't be estimated and a guess of .5 is used as the conservative choice, 95 percent confidence will result in the following accuracy for each sample size:

$$
\begin{array}{rl}
100 & = \pm \ 10\% \ (.10) \\
400 & = \pm \ \ 5\% \ (.05) \\
1,600 & = \pm \ \ 2.5\% \ (.025) \\
6,400 & = \pm \ \ 1.25\% \ (.0125) \\
10,000 & = \pm \ \ 1\% \ (.01)
\end{array}
$$

Where you wish to estimate something that isn't a proportion, such as the number of hospital admissions per typical family practitioner, you first must estimate the standard deviation. This can be done by using a very small sample (e.g., 10) and can be relied on for estimating sample size requirements. Should your original estimate of standard deviation be wrong, you

---

* 2 is used rather than the technically correct 1.96 (for 95 percent confidence) for illustration only, to make calculation easier.

might have to augment your sample later, but it's just as likely to be off in the other direction, meaning the sample would be even larger than needed.

In this example, if you wished to determine the average number of physician-referred admissions per year within ± 10 and your small sample produced a standard deviation of 50, the sample size required for your overall estimate would be:

$$S = \left(\frac{2d}{e} \right)^2$$

d (estimated) $= 50$
e (your choice) $= 10$

$$S = \left(\frac{2 \times 50}{10} \right)^2$$

$$= \frac{100^2}{10}$$

$$= 10^2 = 100$$

If you were willing to take slightly less accuracy, say ± 25, an even smaller sample would do:

$$S = \left(\frac{2d}{e} \right)^2$$

$$= \left(\frac{2 \times 50}{25} \right)^2$$

$$= \left(\frac{100}{25} \right)^2$$

$$= 4^2 = 16$$

This should give you some idea of how useful small, properly drawn samples can be. If you are pragmatic about how precise your estimates must be, and recognize that doubling your precision requires quadrupling your sample, you often will find that small samples do very well.

SURVEY DEVICES

Where you must obtain data directly from people relating to their knowledge, behavior, or attitudes, rather than records, you have basically three choices:

1. mailed questionnaires
2. telephone interviews
3. personal interviews

The mailed questionnaires are likely to be the least expensive per respondent but introduce the greatest chance of self-selection bias in terms of who returns completed forms. Telephone surveys are next in expense, but include some risk of persons' misunderstanding questions, sampling bias against those who don't have phones, and reliance on verbal information. Personal interviews are most expensive but offer chances for observation of respondents and their surroundings, nonverbal clues, etc.

In general, you probably should use a survey research consultant for gathering data from patients and either physicians or the public at large. The use of an outside agency offers both its expertise and its objectivity. Where you ask questions yourself, you must worry lest individuals color their responses in view of who you are. Techniques of question design and objectivity of interviewers are important enough to be left to "experts." Your understanding of the basic process (e.g., sample size requirements) should help you monitor whether your consultants really are expert.

ANALYTICAL OPTIONS

There are a number of useful choices for scaling and analyzing the results from questionnaires and interviews. Some expert consultant advice on the subject would be useful on this subject also. However, there are some specific market research analytical techniques in which you might be interested. One is called importance-performance analysis. In simplest form, it involves asking individuals to indicate what aspects of your behavior or of health services generally are most important to them, then asking them to rate you or other alternatives on each aspect. The results of their responses can be portrayed in a simple matrix showing their rating of important factors on one axis and of performance on the other. Results might look something like that shown in Figure 2-1.

The most satisfactory finding is shown as point B, where you rate well on an important factor. The least satisfactory is point A, where you rate poorly on an important aspect. Point C is poor performance, but in an area unimpor-

Figure 2-1 Importance-Performance Matrix

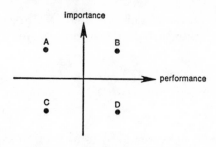

tant to respondents—it may be important to you. Point D represents good performance but in an area not very important to your markets.

This type of analysis can be used to interpret responses by patients, the public at large, physicians on your medical staff or those you'd like to be, employees, board members, and so on. It can be particularly useful in evaluating the results of a market audit. The graphic display (Figure 2-1) is simple enough to be used as a visual aid during presentation and discussion of audit results.

A more sophisticated, quantitative, and complex analytical option is that of conjoint measurement. Such a device is useful in identifying what mix of attributes might be most attractive to a specific market. The technique can be used to measure market preferences among actual competing alternatives or hypothetical options you're using in designing a program. Basically, you ask people to indicate preference for choices with multiple attributes rather than asking about one attribute (e.g., cost, convenience, quality) at a time.

Another technique is trade-off analysis. This approach recognizes that some attributes of choices compete with each other; you can't get more of one without giving up some of the other. Most service options involve some trade-offs, so this mode of analysis is likely to be useful in evaluating program choices from your own point of view as well as from that of your markets. The results of such analysis have been used to predict choices among competing program alternatives and hence to design and modify programs more responsive to market preferences.

The factors that seem to influence choice among health care alternatives by consumers have been identified through numerous studies. They include:

- risk: potential danger from use of services
- convenience: of hours, location, waiting
- cost: monetary, loss of income
- amenities: parking, playroom for children

- personal: physician/employee manner, courtesy, language spoken, cleanliness
- quality: competence, thoroughness, willingness to explain diagnosis, prognosis/therapy

By understanding factors that affect consumer choice, you can employ these kinds of analysis in:

- selecting markets: those whose preferences most closely fit your capacity
- designing services: to match market preferences most closely
- establishing charges: in recognition of how much individuals think your services are worth, rather than how much you know they cost
- deciding where to offer services, at what hours, on which days, etc.
- planning promotion strategies that emphasize what people consider most important and in which you offer superior performance

While most of the examples presented describe analysis of consumer preferences for health service options, the same approaches can be used to examine physician preferences for location of practice or hospital, employee preference for job options or rewards, volunteer choices, donation behavior, etc. By identifying what people are in the market for and seeing options from their perspective, you can decide which markets to aim for and what strategies to use. Examples of employing your understanding of markets in developing strategies are discussed in Chapters 6 and 7 and in the cases in Part IV.

RESEARCH RESULTS

The information generated by market research should be useful in making marketing decisions but never will guarantee success. The more you deal with future realities and anticipated behavior, rather than past or present, the more uncertainty you necessarily introduce. Moreover, the reactions of your competitors to your own marketing efforts are especially difficult to estimate. It is at least a safe assumption, however, that the more you understand about behavior and motivation of patients, physicians, or other organizations, the better you can predict, influence, and respond appropriately to them.

SUMMARY

The process of research involves five steps: (1) identifying decision(s) to be made, (2) determining what you want to know in order to make the best decision(s), (3) designing the appropriate analysis for producing what you want to learn, (4) specifying data needed for such analysis, and (5) designing and executing data collection to generate the appropriate data. This deductive process is designed to ensure that the data you get in Step 5 will be exactly what is most useful in actually making the decision(s) at issue.

The kinds of data necessary for a market audit or as part of developing any particular market strategy cover the same categories: behavior, impacts, causal factors, environment, and competition. The purpose of doing research in these areas is to understand and later predict, influence, and respond to how individuals and organizations will behave.

The effective collection of data in market research requires identification of the population of interest, determining the sample size and sampling method to be used, deciding how to obtain facts or feelings from the sample, and scaling or otherwise preparing the responses for analysis. Small samples provide useful insights, and the precise sample size required can be calculated from a simple formula. Expert advice and the help of consultants in designing and executing market research is recommended for both their technical competence and their objectivity.

Analytical methods useful in examining choice behavior include importance-performance analysis, conjoint measurement, and trade-off analysis. These techniques can be used in identifying your own preferences as well as those of your markets. Specific analyses can be made as part of market selection, service design, location and price decisions, or promotional strategy development. Each enables the organization to quantify market preference for multiple and even competing attributes of actual or hypothetical choices.

Readings

Preference Factors

Hetherington, R., and Hopkins, C. "Symptom Sensitivity: Its Social and Cultural Correlates." *Health Services Research,* Spring 1969, p. 63.

Howard, J., et al. "Humanizing Health Care—The Implications of Technology, Centralization and Self-Care." *Medical Care* 1515, Supplement, May 1977, p. 11.

Metzner, C., and Bashshur, R. "Factors Associated with Choice of Health Care Plans." *Journal of Health and Social Behavior* 8, 1967, p. 291.

Scitovsky, A., et al. "Factors Affecting the Choice Between Two Prepaid Plans." *Medical Care* 16:8, August 1978, p. 660.

Steele, J. "Conceptual and Empirical Dimensions of Health Behavior." *Journal of Health and Social Behavior* 13, December 1972, p. 382.

Stratmann, W. "A Study of Consumer Attitudes About Health Care: The Delivery of Ambulatory Services." *Medical Care* 13:7, July 1975, p. 537.

Ware, J., and Snyder, M. "Dimensions of Patient Attitudes Regarding Doctors and Medical Care Services." *Medical Care* 13:8, August 1975, p. 669.

Physician Behavior

Anderson, N. "Looking for Configurality in Clinical Judgment." *Psychological Bulletin* 78, August 1972, p. 93.

Creditor, M.C., and V.K. "The Ecology of an Urban Voluntary Hospital: The Referral Chain." *Medical Care* 10:1, January-February 1972, p. 88.

Fryzel, R. "Marketing Nonprofit Institutions." *Hospital and Health Services Administration* 23:1, Winter 1978, p. 8.

Johnson, A.C., et al. "The Office Practice of Internists III: Characteristics of Patients." *JAMA* 193, 1965, p. 916.

Kirkwood, C.W. *Decision Analysis Incorporating Preferences of Groups,* Ph.D. dissertation. Cambridge, Mass.: Massachusetts Institute of Technology, 1972.

Tanaka, A. "Problems Facing Rural Physicians: Do the Boondocks *Really* Need Docs?" *Federation Bulletin* 65:1, January 1978, p. 3.

Data Collection

Flexner, W., et al. "Discovering What the Health Consumer Really Wants." *Health Care Management Review* 2:4, Fall 1977, p. 43.

Goldman, A. "The Group Depth Interview." *Journal of Marketing* 26, 1962, p. 61.

Leonard, D. "Can Focus Group Interviews Survive?" *Marketing News* 9, October 10, 1975, p. 6.

Importance-Performance

Martilla, J., and Carvey, D. "Four Subtle Sins in Marketing Research." *Journal of Marketing* 39:1, January 1975, p. 10.

Martilla, J., and James, J. "Importance-Performance Analysis." *Journal of Marketing* 41:1, January 1977, p. 77.

Myers, J., and Alpers, M. "Determining Attributes: Meaning and Measurement." *Journal of Marketing* 32:4, October 1968, p. 13.

Swan, J., and Coombs, L.J. "Product Performance and Consumer Satisfaction: A New Concept." *Journal of Marketing* 40:2, April 1976, p. 25.

Conjoint Measurement

Ford, D.L., et al. "Predicting Job Choices with Models That Contain Subjective Probability Judgments: An Empirical Comparison of Five Models." *Organizational Behavior & Human Performance* 7, 1972, p. 397.

Green, P., et al. "Benefit Bundle Analysis." *Journal of Advertising Research* 12, 1972, p. 31.

Green, P., and Wind, Y. "New Way to Measure Consumer's Judgment", *Harvard Business Review* 53, 1975, p. 107.

Koutsopoulos, K., et al. "Psychometric Modeling of Consumer Decisions in Primary Health Care." *Health Services Research* 12:4, Winter 1977, p. 427.

Wind, Y, and Spitz, L. "Analytical Approach to Marketing Decisions in Health-Care Organizations." *Operations Research* 24:5, September-October 1976, p. 973.

Trade-Off Analysis

Fischhoff, B., et al. "How Safe Is Safe Enough? A Psychometric Study of Attitudes Toward Technological Risks and Benefits." *Policy Sciences* 9:2, April 1978, p. 127.

Grimes, R., et al. "Use of Decision Theory in Regional Planning." *Health Services Research* 9:1, Spring 1974, p. 58.

Johnson, R. "Trade-off Analysis of Consumer Values." *Journal of Marketing Research* 11, 1974, p. 121.

McClain J., and Rao, V. "Trade-offs and Conflicts in Evaluation of Health System Alternatives: Methodology for Analysis." *Health Services Research* 9:1, Spring 1974, p. 35.

Parker, B., and Srinivasan, V. "A Consumer Preference Approach to the Planning of Rural Primary Health Care Facilities." *Operations Research* 24:5, September-October 1976, p. 991.

Research Results

Acito, F. "Consumer Decision-Making and Health Maintenance Organizations: A Review." *Medical Care* 16:1, January 1978, p. 1.

Brooks, C. "Associations Among Distance, Patient Satisfaction and Utilization of Two Types of Inner-City Clinics." *Medical Care,* September/October 1973, p. 62.

Houston, C., and Pasanen, W. "Patients' Perceptions of Hospital Care." *Hospitals, JAHA* 46, 1972, p. 70.

Hulka, B., et al. "Correlates of Satisfaction and Dissatisfaction with Medical Care: A Community Perspective." *Medical Care* 13, 1975, p. 648.

Lebow, J. "Consumer Assessments of the Quality of Medical Care." *Medical Care* 12, 1974, p. 328.

Marshall, C., et al. "Time and Distance in Rural Practice: Dissatisfaction with Travel Distance to the Physician in a Rural Area." *Journal of the Kansas Medical Society* 70, 1969, p. 93.

Chapter 3
Market Audit/ Research Output

There are three major outputs of the market audit/market research process:

1. identification of problems
2. identification of threats
3. identification of opportunities

All three are related to two factors: changes in behavior and action decisions. For purposes of discussion, the three terms will be defined as follows:

1. Problem: a current situation or trend that, unless changed, will damage the organization's mission or health significantly (if it hasn't already). A problem implies the necessity of taking action to alter deliberately what the future would be without your intervention.
2. Threat: a potential situation whose occurrence is by no means certain, but is of sufficient likelihood to justify your concern. A threat implies the necessity of your intervention to *avoid* a change that otherwise might occur.
3. Opportunity: a potential situation whose occurrence is by no means certain, but is of sufficient attractiveness to you to justify taking advantage of it. An opportunity implies the desirability of your intervention to achieve a change that will benefit your community, your organization, and, it is hoped, both.

The key factors in distinguishing the three outcomes are the positive vs. negative aspects of a situation and its present vs. future existence. A problem is a negative situation in the present that will continue or become worse in the future unless you act. A threat is a negative situation that might exist in the future unless you act. An opportunity is a positive current situation that you can improve into the future by acting. The labels are not important in themselves. Each requires that you act so as to achieve or prevent a change in outcomes; each requires that you achieve or prevent a change in behavior.

PROBLEMS

A problem may be identified in any of the five audit categories: impact, behavior, causal factors, environment, and competition. Low occupancy, idle capacity, net operating losses, fiscal overextension, inadequate reserves, and unacceptable morbidity or mortality all are examples of problems in impact. Each can be understood as resulting from some combination of behaviors. Either overbuilding or low admission rates may explain low occupancy, depending on your perspective. High receivables may result from slow processing of payments by third party reimbursement organizations, slow payment by patients, or slow processing of bills by your business office.

Unacceptable mortality or morbidity may be viewed as entirely *their* fault: resulting from excessive smoking, drinking, drug abuse, unsafe driving, poor nutrition, or some other of their behaviors. It also may be seen as the result of *your* behavior: failure to provide information, education, or guidance; failure to offer sufficient incentives for *them* to change their behavior. Ascribing blame is likely to serve little purpose however. If you see your mission as improving health, then somehow you have to act to get them to change their behavior. Chances are this will require you to change something about your behavior.

A classic example of how the same outcome could result from differences in behavior is the commonplace low occupancy in obstetrics units. In any given situation, such low occupancy could result from specific behaviors by the patient population:

- decline in fertility rate among women
- tendencies to prefer home delivery or birth centers to hospital obstetrics units
- greater use of contraceptives
- increasing preference for abortions rather than delivery as the outcome of pregnancy

Exactly whose behavior (market segments such as older or younger women, affluent vs. poor, white vs. nonwhite, primiparous vs. multiparous mothers) is causing the low occupancy may make a difference in whether or how you approach the problem.

The same situation could be caused by behavior of physicians:

- failure of a sufficient number of obstetricians, or other physicians practicing obstetrics, to join your medical staff
- tendency by those physicians on your staff to refer a significant number of admissions to another hospital

Your approach to these situations clearly would be different since one reflects physicians *not* on your staff and the other relates to physicians who are.

This same situation could be viewed as resulting from your behavior. You may have expanded your obstetrics unit recently in the mistaken belief that fertility rates would increase or remain high, or that more physicians practicing obstetrics would join your staff, or that your market share would increase. Since occupancy is the ratio of your census to your bed supply, their behavior can only be related to census; your behavior is responsible for bed supply. Your behavior also may be involved if you have failed to provide the equipment, facilities, staff, or amenities to attract or retain medical staff or patients.

Problems also may be identified among causal factors. Shifts in population numbers, age, sex, income, or residence may be viewed as a problem if their effects on behavior and impacts are negative. A decrease in the number of women of childbearing age could be the reason for low obstetrics census, independent of fertility rates. Preference for small families or wishes to have careers may explain lower fertility rates. Changes in psychographics and in individuals' attitudes about their health, their behavior, or you, also may be considered problems.

Externalities also may be considered problems. Changes in the local economy may have produced lower ability to pay costs of health care, or lower use of services, or both. High unemployment may have forced many wives to look for work and caused a reduction in fertility. Shifts in policy by government or other third party payers may have produced financial problems without changes in utilization. Since identifying a situation as a problem implies your intention to change it, you must be sure that external factors identified as problems are subject to your effective intervention. If you can't change the local economy or government policies, you'll have to look elsewhere for a strategy.

The competition certainly may be considered a problem for many organizations. "Raiding" of employees, physicians, or patients is a fairly common allegation. Duplication of a service you offer may be viewed as a problem by local planning agencies as well as by you. Competitors' price reductions, in contrast, may be a problem to you but a boon to planning agencies and consumers. Perhaps uniquely in the health field, you have the option of cooperating with your competition to reduce or eliminate mutual problems for the public good, subject, of course, to a careful look at possible antitrust implications. Unless you can expect to alter a competitor's behavior of course, you shouldn't define it as a problem, but merely accept it as a constraining or complicating factor in the environment. Where you can alter such behavior, your competition may be targeted for change much like your markets.

Examples

Some examples of problems that cut across categories and demonstrate the dynamic interaction of the audit factors include:

- overuse of hospital emergency rooms because of insurance company exclusion of office visits (environment); physicians' not having office hours during evenings, weekends, or holidays (behavior); preference for fully equipped facilities (psychographics) or inability of poor minorities to attract physicians to their communities (demographics/psychographics); the impact on the community in higher cost of care or long waits for service and the resulting dissatisfaction

- avoidance of immunizations by families for their school-age children due to low levels of concern over risks of polio or measles (psychographics), or difficulty in getting appointments (behavior) with resulting higher incidence of preventable disease (impact)

- proliferation of Medicaid and abortion "mills" (competition) resulting in increased government regulation (environment) bringing with it excessive recordkeeping requirements for you (behavior), higher costs and a poorer financial situation (impact)

The key to effective problem identification in the market audit is to be thorough in portraying and understanding the causal relationships across the factors and to be precise in identifying where you intend to intervene. A problem is a situation you intend to change, so you must be sure you're prepared to change whatever causal factor, behavior, or impact you label a problem. Since most problems result from an interaction of your behavior and that of one of your markets, you always have the choice of changing your own behavior rather than theirs. Your options are discussed in Chapters 6 and 7.

THREATS

Threats also may be identified in any one of the five audit categories. Any foreseeable potential change in environment, competition, causal factors, behavior, or impact that would cause damage if it occurred is a threat. By labeling such a foreseeable development a threat, you indicate your determination to avoid it. The extent of the threat should be measured both in terms of its probability of occurrence and its consequences (impact) if it did occur.

A potentially damaging change in behavior is most likely to be identified as a threat. One or more physicians who are likely to retire, cut back their practice, or leave the area can be viewed as a threat by the hospital where they are on the medical staff or by the community they serve. The age of your medical staff members and their expressed intentions may be used to gauge the probability of this threat. The number of admissions or referrals each physician has provided in the past may help you evaluate the consequences.

A classic example of a behavioral threat is that of the hospital with significant dependence on a major market that soon may seek care elsewhere. If your hospital now gets 25 percent of its admissions from an area that sends you 50 percent of its admissions, you would be delighted. If that area begins talking about developing its own hospital or competing program, you would see the same situation as a threat.

Demographic and psychographic factors also are potential threats. Foreseeable shifts in population location, age, sex, or insurance coverage could represent the threat of significant changes in behavior. Only where such changes could be prevented or their consequences in impact averted would they serve as a focus for strategy development, however. An example might be a shift toward preference for birth centers for routine obstetric deliveries. Rather than be damaged by such a shift, a hospital could develop its own birth center to accommodate changes in preference rather than curse the decline in obstetrics admissions.

Environmental factors could threaten damage to your organization's health or mission. National health insurance, regulated cost containment "caps," or technology that makes some services obsolete would represent threats to specific organizations. The advent of Dr. Jonas Salk's polio vaccine was a definite threat to the March of Dimes and Sister Kenny Foundations. Whether such threats can be foreseen and whether they can or should be avoided is a question of values and competence for each organization.

A potential action by a competitor is likely to be a threat. A classic example would be a competitor's seeking a certificate of need to duplicate a service you now offer that is barely capable of holding its own. There are a number of examples in hospital primary care development where one institution singled out an area that had been without medical care for years, only to discover a second institution working on developing a similar program in the same place. Again, whether you can and should act to forestall or prevent the negative impact of a competitive threat is a matter of both values and competence.

Examples

One example might be the previously cited case of a hospital that gets a large share of its patients from a community that never had a hospital. As the community grows and referrals to the hospital also grow, so does the threat that the community will develop its own institution to improve access to care and enhance local pride. If the existing institution develops a satellite program in that community, beginning with primary and emergency care and perhaps adding long-term and eventually acute inpatient care, the wishes of the community and health of the hospital both may be served.

Another possible threat is the emphasis on regionalization and concentration of specialized services. While such developments represent opportunities to larger hospitals, for example, they may constitute threats to smaller ones. If unable to compete effectively for physicians by offering comparable equipment, smaller rural hospitals may have difficulty maintaining viability. If pressed to reduce bed supplies or increase occupancy by regulatory agencies, smaller institutions may find it hard to avoid delaying or turning away admissions, and may be at a competitive disadvantage vs. large hospitals.

Similarly, the single service organization may be at a competitive disadvantage against its more comprehensive counterpart. An organization that offers multiple interventions for a specific health problem has a distinct advantage over one that has only a single "solution" (see Chapter 14). Threats that publicly subsidized programs may begin competing with private, and gain a price advantage, are another real possibility. Hospitals that open primary care centers may threaten private practitioners through offering more comprehensive "one-stop" services, including laboratory and x-ray, or by offering charges covered by health insurance, or both.

Since threats require attention, care must be taken in labeling foreseeable situations as threats. The importance of a threat as a target for your intervention should be evaluated according to three criteria:

1. the probability that the threatening event or development will be realized in the future
2. the severity of the impact that event or development will have on the organization's mission or viability
3. the probability of the organization's successfully averting or accommodating the event or development if it does occur

Whether these criteria are applied through formal quantitative analysis, through informal group processes, or intuition is a matter for the organization to judge. Some preliminary intuition about the seriousness of the threat will be needed even to decide how much time and attention to devote to analyzing it. In any case, the effective manager should be able to identify and distinguish the importance of different threats and ultimately to act to avert or minimize them. Specific marketing strategies for averting threats are discussed in Chapter 6 and a case example of unsuccessful treatment of threats in Chapter 18.

OPPORTUNITIES

The distinction between an opportunity and a problem may be small and relatively academic in practice. Both are situations you target for change. The chief distinction is the extent to which you feel compelled to achieve a change rather than merely to desire it. For an ambitious, growing organization, this distinction may be exceedingly small. In any case, the focus of attention is the same: on the possibility of changing a situation for the better.

Behavioral opportunities are the chief area for attention in the market audit results. All opportunities can be viewed in terms of positive changes in behavior that are possible, just as threats are negative changes in behavior that are avoidable, and problems are positive changes in behavior that are necessary. The typical market opportunities consist of three classes of behavioral changes:

1. getting more customers for your present services or opening up new markets for current products
2. getting current customers to use new services or new products for existing markets
3. attracting new customers for new services or new products for new markets

The typical health organization may tend to think of these opportunities in terms of its own behavior: offering new services or developing new markets. The key to the marketing approach, however, is the realization that successful changes in your program are dependent on getting people to use your new or expanded services, not merely on developing or expanding your capacity. For some services, especially inpatient or emergency care, the consumer may have little choice but to use those prescribed, but even there you will have to attract the physicians, regulatory approvals, and staff to provide the services successfully. Where customers have more options as to whether or where to seek care, you are more dependent on their choice and should focus more attention on predicting and influencing their behavior.

A behavioral opportunity is simply a situation where there is an apparent prospect that people will use your services who didn't before (new markets) or use services you didn't offer before (new products) or perhaps choose you more frequently as the source of a regular service. To take advantage of these opportunities will involve increasing the size of your market, your share of existing markets, or both.

Your analysis of markets and market shares may indicate opportunities. What you are looking for is an area or segment where you would expect a larger share and where the market is of substantial size. Residents of the surrounding community would be a typical example. If your share of the services they use is small, and that of an organization farther away is large, you should start by considering the situation an opportunity. In effect, you have a natural competitive advantage (proximity) that is not reflected in your market share. If you can discover the reason why people choose the farther alternative, and correct it, you should anticipate your natural advantage to be effective. (It should be recognized that your opportunities are, in effect, threats to your competitors in many cases.)

An opportunity often will be apparent from analysis of your performance (impact). The best kinds of new service to develop are those most closely akin to those you now offer that you are performing well. If you are succeeding at offering family planning services, you might add genetics counseling to expand the comprehensiveness of your programs to the same population. Good performance tells you that you're doing something right, and analysis may reveal that the same approach would work elsewhere. Such analysis should be done carefully, however. There is an unfortunate tendency to assume that where a program succeeds, its design and execution were self-evidently perfect and worthy of repetition. An example of this, together with its shortcomings, is presented in Chapter 14.

Analysis of demographic and psychographic information also may reveal an opportunity. Increasing numbers of persons with characteristics especially suited to your programs may well signal the prospect of increasing utilization. Changes in preference may be an opportunity if you can alter your programs in the direction preferences are moving. Growing awareness of a health problem or of the availability of a treatment for it may occur naturally in the community or be enhanced by your own communications efforts. If you couple such a trend with an offering of the treatment, or expanding your current offering, you should be in a position to benefit your organization as well as the community.

In marketing, the assumption almost always is made that a problem, threat, or opportunity for you is *always* an opportunity for the community.

Since you will have to improve the benefits individuals derive to get them to change their behavior, they are, by definition, better off. With increasing third party payment for health services, of course, whether they are sufficiently better off to warrant the overall increase in health expenditures that results is a matter of communitywide and nationwide concern.

A well-known example of this issue is the promotional effort by Sunrise Hospital in Las Vegas. By offering patients who are admitted on Friday or Saturday a chance on a drawing for a two-week, all-expense-paid cruise for two, the hospital has been able to change behavior toward evening out its census variation from weekday to weekend and attracting more patients. Clearly, the patients benefit: they enjoy the added chance for a free cruise. The hospital benefits by achieving greater occupancy and efficiency. Whether the costs to the community for hospital care change for the better is the ultimate test of whether this is a "successful" marketing effort, from the community's rather than the hospital's or patient's perspective.

Opportunities may derive from developments in the environment. Certificate of need, for example, tends to limit competition and concentrate specialized services. In one case, a hospital designated as the only source of Level III neonatal intensive care in its region had an immediate opportunity to become the major obstetrics hospital because of the wishes of increasing numbers of obstetricians to practice there. Recognizing when such developments give you a new market advantage can be key to your success.

Even competitors may represent an opportunity now and then. Those of their programs that are failing may end up opening new markets for you. Their dissatisfied medical staff or patients may be ready to turn to you. You may attempt to take advantage of such opportunities by open warfare in the spirit of cutthroat competition or work in cooperation with other organizations to foster more effective mutual market developments (see Chapter 9). Increasing pressures that threaten the survival of marginal programs and organizations necessarily represent opportunities for those that survive.

Examples

Some classic examples of opportunities are medically underserved areas. Both rural and urban communities exist that have been unable to attract and retain permanent sources of medical care. Substantial subsidies are available to organizations that propose to develop services in such areas. The Health in Underserved Rural Areas (HURA), Rural Health Initiatives (RHI), and Robert Wood Johnson Foundation rural primary care development programs are examples for rural areas. Through the Department of Housing and Urban Development (HUD) and the Johnson foundation, primary care group practice subsidies have been available for urban areas.

Such opportunities are not guaranteed, of course. In assessing an opportunity such as an area lacking an obviously "needed" service, your organization should ask why no such offering has developed or succeeded. It may be that the area's residents simply don't use the service, are perfectly happy with an existing source somewhere else, or can't pay for it. Assuming such areas automatically are ripe for the picking can be a mistake, as is described in Chapter 15.

The government's emphasis on reducing excess hospital capacity and on inpatient care utilization represents a substantial opportunity for alternative program developments. Such obvious alternatives as ambulatory surgery, long-term and home care already are well under way in many communities. If they are not in yours, you might look into them. Other health-related interests in the community involving weight control, stop-smoking clinics, positive wellness, or holistic health represent other possible areas for future development. While the extent of third party insurance coverage for such services is minimal now, it may grow if promised effects on reducing expensive medical care utilization are realized.

There is a legend to the effect that Napoleon's mother invested all her extra money in British war bonds. While disloyal on the surface, her reasoning was faultless and prescient. She figured that the only country that could topple her son from power would be Great Britain, so by investing in British war bonds, she was covered whoever won. Similarly, hospitals may wish to hedge their bets by becoming their own competition, developing ambulatory care alternatives or successors to their current inpatient programs. Where their reputations are strong and backup services are comprehensive, hospitals should enjoy a competitive advantage over single-service alternatives.

The important point to keep in mind about a market opportunity is that it is found in the potential willingness of the public—the customers—to change how they behave. You must be willing to design and execute changes in your own programs that meet the public's expectations in order to take advantage of such opportunities. The kinds of opportunities coming along in the future will be chiefly those involving high degrees of consumer choice, so this marketing reality is becoming increasingly important.

SUMMARY

The three outputs of the market audit are problems, threats, and opportunities. Problems are existing situations that make you so uncomfortable you feel you must change them. Threats are potential future situations whose prospect makes you so uncomfortable you feel you must avoid them. Opportunities are existing or potential situations that would make you feel a lot more comfortable if you took advantage of them. All three require a strategy for change, either to achieve or to prevent an alteration in the way some market behaves with respect to you.

Problems, threats, and opportunities may be found in any of the five areas examined in the market audit: impact, behavior, causes, environment, or competition. As in all marketing efforts, however, the focus of attention must be on behavior: yours, your market's, external organization's, or your competition's. You must determine whether you can change or merely predict and anticipate such behavior. How much time and effort you devote to such efforts will be determined on the basis of three factors: what changes are most threatening or promising, which are most likely, and which you can most effectively do something about.

Problems, threats, and opportunities are merely labels to help you analyze market audit results systematically. An opportunity for you is potentially a threat to your competition. A problem for you may be an opportunity for your competition. Whether you deal with problems, threats, and opportunities in a competitive, empire-building or a cooperative, public-spirited way is one of the major marketing choices uniquely available to health care organizations.

Two important pieces of information should come out of your market audit: identification of your major markets and determination of your market shares in each market. This would be displayed in a matrix such as is shown in Exhibit 3-1.

Your market segmentation may follow any groupings that help you distinguish different populations and for whom you can get service utilization information. Some useful examples would be residence of markets (zip codes, census tracts, cities/counties), referring or admitting physician, and patient categories (diagnosis, source of payment, age). When done by residence or other population characteristics, this analysis tells you your major service

---

Exhibit 3-1 Market Problems, Threats, and Opportunities in Market Shares

Market Segment	Number of Service Uses: Your Organization	Percent of All Your Uses	Number of Their Uses: Any Organization	Percent Yours= Market Share
A	400	20	600	66.7
B	200	10	800	25
C	600	30	800	75
D	300	15	600	50
E	500	25	2,000	25
	2,000	100	4,800	41.7

areas or populations and what proportion of the total business you get. When performed for physicians or referral agencies, it tells you upon which providers you are most dependent, major admitters (referrers), and how much they depend on you (shares).

In this example, segments A and C are giving you a substantial proportion of their business and there is little opportunity for growth. They may be threats, however, if competition should make inroads there. Segments B and E suggest opportunities for growth, but E offers greater promise because of its size. Whether any or all of these segments constitute problems depends on their specific impacts: percentage who pay, follow advice, keep appointments, etc. Such additional information will focus your efforts further on whichever segments merit greatest attention.

Market segment/market share analysis should be done for as many segments and services as you can find time and data. The results of such analysis when performed initially will identify precisely where your attention is warranted and is likely to prove worthwhile. The results of repeated periodic analyses will reveal precisely where your marketing efforts have succeeded or failed and enable you to modify your efforts in the future. Marketing without such data is the equivalent of flying without radar. By chance alone, you'll succeed some of the time, but your failures may be disastrous.

Chapter 4

Managing the Audit Process

Having described the technical and analytical aspects of carrying out a market audit, it is time to discuss the practical management aspects. Since marketing itself is not an altogether accepted discipline in health care, primarily because of misunderstanding, the market audit may seem a prelude to improperly manipulating public thought and behavior. With its focus on the collection of information rather than manipulating behavior, however, the audit should be an acceptable starting point in most health organizations. The kinds of data collected and analysis applied are not that dissimilar from traditional planning and management data bases.

Because a market audit potentially includes an endless array of information, and because of the limited familiarity most organizations have with the audit process, it makes sense to introduce the market audit incrementally. This nose-under-the-tent or foot-in-the-door strategy is itself a marketing technique, part of your marketing of a marketing program (see Chapter 12). Since marketing means identifying and responding to the perceived or awakened needs, wants, and desires of your markets, you should treat the market audit as a potential product, representing your response.

In effect, this means that the market audit should respond to the knowledge, beliefs, and attitudes of those within your organization who will participate in the audit process and use its results. Such a participative design process for the audit should smooth the way for its acceptance and promote the use of its results. In allowing participation by others, you will lose some control over the design, but this should be more than compensated for by improved prospects of acceptance and use. In most institutions, the important step will be to get agreement on and cooperation in the market audit process, independent of its specific content. Technical improvements can be carried out once the basic idea is accepted.

There is an alternative strategy for winning acceptance of the market audit that can be mentioned, though not recommended by the author. This is the whole camel or door-in-the-face technique that suggests you ask people for much more than you really expect to get, anticipating their refusal, then back off to your real wishes later. The idea behind this technique is that consistently refusing diminishing requests makes people uncomfortable, and at some point they'll give in. However, this is a clearly manipulative strategy and is likely to yield grudging rather than wholehearted cooperation.

On the assumption that a foot-in-the-door approach is preferred, and group participation more effective than individual edict, the design of the market audit can take advantage of a number of group processes. Formal techniques such as Nominal Group may be used to identify specific items of content for the audit. A procedure such as the following would be suggested:

1. Gather together the individuals who should participate in the market audit design. Divide them into groups of six to eight, seated around tables in the same room but sufficiently far from each other that one group's discussions don't interfere with other groups. Describe in detail the specific procedures to be followed (as outlined here) and identify the time frames for their accomplishment. Make sure the persons understand and accept the "rules" of Nominal Group that outlaw discussion much of the time and control interaction quite rigidly.

2. Distribute cards or pieces of paper and pens or pencils to each participant. Ask each participant to write down personal suggestions for audit content, divided into two parts each time. When listing impact factors, half the time should be spent on impacts the organization has on its community (outcomes) and half on impacts the community has on the organization (performance). When listing behavior, half the time should be spent on the organization's, half on those of the markets; for causes, half on demographic, half on psychographic; on externalities, half on environment and half on the competition.

3. Total time spent in writing down ideas on one specific subject should be limited to 10 or 15 minutes. When the time is up, participants will be instructed to go on to the next subject—turn over their paper or use another piece. Two subjects or parts at a time can be handled most easily. Upon completion of the jotting down of ideas, group discussion can begin.

4. Discussion should be controlled by a moderator for each group who asks each individual member, in turn, to report on one suggestion. The moderator records this on a large board or series of sheets for future reference. Not until all the suggestions are recorded is any discussion or evaluation allowed.

5. Once all the ideas are recorded, the group is encouraged to discuss, evaluate, and reach consensus about what are the most important items to include in the market audit. The items should be specific pieces of information desired, not questions to be asked or processes of analysis to be followed. The answers or specific facts and feelings the organization wants most to discover should be the starting point for audit design. Specification of survey and analytical methodology can be carried out independently (Chapter 2).

Brainstorming or other group discussions also may be used to identify market audit content. The Nominal Group Technique is especially useful where individuals are unfamiliar with each other, or where some would tend to dominate group discussions because of formal or informal positions of power. The act of using a group process rather than an outside expert or executive fiat is likely to ensure that the audit will be useful and used.

INSIDE/OUTSIDE AUDITS

For purposes of understanding and implementing a market audit, it can be thought of as encompassing two separable parts: an inside audit and an outside version. The inside audit focuses on the specific market segments with which the organization currently has market relationships: active patients, medical staff, referring agencies, etc. The external audit, by contrast, covers market segments with which the organization might be expected, now or in the foreseeable future, to have market relationships: nonpatients in your service area, physicians who don't admit or refer patients, or referral agencies that might but don't use you.

The inside audit may be preferred as a starting point for two reasons. First, it is easier to carry out since most of the data will be in your own records or come from persons with whom you have some contact. Second, the results of the inside audit will be more self-evidently important and meaningful and can be used to design a focused external audit later. Once the internal audit identifies what problems, threats, and opportunities pertain to your current markets, you can use the external audit to help develop effective strategies for reaching new markets or developing new services, if necessary.

The limitations of the inside audit should be recognized at the outset, however. Whenever you examine your current markets' behavior, demographics, or psychographics (and how the environment or competition affect *them*), you're dealing with a potentially biased self-selected sample of the entire market. Each market segment you analyze differs from the whole in at least one important respect: it chose to seek care from *your* organization.

Therefore, you cannot assume that its characteristics, feelings, or behavior are representative of everyone.

To find out why you may have been losing patients or physicians, for example, you might not get all the answers you need by asking patients or physicians you've kept. They must be somewhat different from those who were lost, or all would have been lost or all would have stayed. To be sure you know who was lost and why, you'd have to survey those you lost. Similarly, if you wish to attract new markets, you can't be sure your present customers are representative of those who aren't doing business with you. Only an external audit will yield reliable data on persons with whom you don't have market relations.

The costs and difficulties of an external audit are likely to be much greater than for an internal one. The kinds of data you wish to collect and the facts and feelings you need to discover are essentially the same, however. You want to learn how your noncustomers behave, their demographic and psychographic attributes, how they affect your competition, how your competition behaves toward them, and how environmental factors affect them. Since your noncustomers potentially are a much larger group than your present customers, and since you can't rely on your own records or contacts to produce needed data, it makes sense to focus your external audit.

By identifying problems, threats, and opportunities through an internal audit, you should be able to determine exactly the external markets in which you're most interested. By determining which problems, threats, and opportunities are most promising or dangerous, you can rank potential new markets accordingly. Specific techniques for priority ranking are discussed in Chapter 8.

Like the internal audit, the external version is likely to be a halting, incomplete, and error-prone effort at first. It, too, should improve over time as experience is gained with the procedure and results. As the outputs of both internal and external audits prove useful to the organization in planning market strategies and evaluating their results, the level of interest in and support for the audit will improve. Most health organizations have the time to learn through trial and error. The perfect, all-purpose audit probably does not exist, and can't.

GENERAL VS. SPECIFIC

In addition to the inside vs. outside alternatives for the market audit, there are choices regarding general or specific content and analysis. Given the virtually endless number of possible market segments, environmental factors, or competitors you might examine, and the equally endless amount of detail you might seek about each, an audit could become a career rather than a contained effort. At the outset, in getting your feet wet, it would be prudent to deal with many factors generally, then move on to specifics.

Market segments, for example, can be established based on a virtually infinite number of factors. You could divide your geographic region into counties, cities, towns, zip codes, census tracts, blocks, and even block faces if you wish. Only you can decide how precisely you want to identify different markets, recognizing the costs and potential benefits of increasingly detailed analysis. In the first go-round, at least, a more general analysis may be useful unless you have reason to suspect strongly that there are specific geographic differences among small areas.

Similarly, segments based on age, ethnicity, income levels, etc., may be broken into many very small groupings rather than a few large ones. Here again, greater specificity may be useful in measuring impact, behavior, or psychographics. Health status measures, especially, should be made on population subgroups (e.g., infant mortality for whites vs. nonwhites, urban vs. rural). Factors that have a known influence on use of services (race, income, age, sex) should be reflected in analysis, though separate segments may not be maintained for each.

A first general, then specific, rule can be followed as the market audit is introduced, much like the first inside, then outside. Where problems, threats, and opportunities appear in a general analysis, more specific breakdowns can follow, focusing on the details of what was found in the general analysis. There is a risk in this approach, of course. There may be some specific problems, threats, and opportunities that are masked by a general analysis. A lack of overall population growth may hide a rise in women of childbearing age or the over-65 age group. General population growth may mask a decline in a specific age, ethnic, or geographic segment you serve. Only good management intuition can draw the line as to where more general analysis is warranted (as opposed to risky, or more specific analysis) vs. overly expensive.

PRESENT VS. FUTURE

The third continuum in developing first vs. subsequent versions of the market audit is that of time frame. An audit is incomplete if it merely covers the present. Looking at current behavior, impacts, and causal factors is taking a still picture of a dynamic situation. You really want to know what aspects of the situation are fine now but getting worse, or bad now but getting better without your intervention. To know how things are going in the full sense of the word, you have to know the direction and rate of change in which they're moving as well as where they are right now.

A number of forecasting techniques are available to anticipate where general or specific situations are going. Which you use should depend on how important the situation is to you, how sensitive your decisions would be to its changes, and how feasible it is for you to use more complex vs. simpler alternatives. Here, too, you can follow an incremental approach, using simpler techniques as a screening device to identify critical changes, then more complex and thorough analysis to focus specifically on those critical situations.

Trend analysis is a common approach to forecasting. Even in your first market audit, you may employ past trends if you can collect data on the measures you're using for the past as well as the present. Past health status measures, census and occupancy levels, financial statements, medical records on patient behavior, census data, and perhaps even some prior survey results may be available. Wherever you have measured the same element in the past, you should be able at least to identify a trend.

There are three basic techniques for trend analysis: extrapolation and simple and multiple correlation. Extrapolation merely portrays the trend in the past, either graphically or mathematically, and projects the trend into the future. Records on past numbers of visits, registrations, census, income, expenditures, etc., may be used for trend extrapolation. The basic flaw in this technique is its unquestioned assumption that past trends necessarily will continue into the future. Such an assumption is easy to make, but dangerous. Unless you understand why past trends have occurred and are confident that they will continue in the same direction at the same rate, there is no particularly good reason to project a continuing trend as opposed to no change or a reversal.

Instead of merely accepting and projecting a past trend without understanding it, you can tie that trend to changes in a second factor. Past utilization changes may be explained by population changes and the link established through a use rate. Use rates themselves may have changed in the past due to the aging of the population. Your hospital admissions may be related directly to the number of physicians on your staff and their admissions rates. By identifying a single factor strongly linked to the specific impact, behavior, or causal factor you're predicting, you have at least attempted to understand why past changes have occurred and link future changes to an explanatory factor.

The risk in trend correlation is that more than one factor may be responsible for past trends and important to future developments. Admission rates may alter with the age of the population as well as the size of the medical staff, or the staff members' specialties rather than merely their numbers. Health status should change logically as the result of changes in environmental hazards, how individuals care for their own health, and the evolution of a complex set of health services, rather than your specific program. Using a single factor may make forecasting simple but can risk overlooking the effects of other important factors.

There are specific techniques of multivariate analysis that can take into account as many factors as you can identify and measure relative to what you're forecasting. Multiple linear regressions, complex systems dynamics models, and multivariate simulations are among the choices. All tend to be more complex and expensive to use, but try to identify and measure the precise effects of most important factors rather than ignoring them or using only one. For short-term forecasting, they are especially useful. For longer range forecasting, they are dependent on getting forecasts of all the factors, which may involve making a lot of wild guesses to come up with one scientific-looking wild guess as a result.

FACTOR FORECASTING

The author recommends an approach called factor forecasting. It is not a quantitative method per se, although it can use the results of quantitative analysis, including any of the trend analyses described previously. It is designed to be used in a group process and to include persons outside as well as within the organization.

The first step in the process is to select the participants. These should include those who are part of designing the market audit but should extend to informed persons in the community who are knowledgeable about what you're forecasting and may be affected by it. Since the purpose of your forecast is to identify where action is needed, those who will be part of and affected by the kinds of action you'd take should be included. The group then uses a formal (e.g., Nominal Group) or informal (brainstorming) process to identify change factors.

The factors identified should meet two important criteria:

1. They should have significant and predictable effects on the element you're forecasting.
2. They should be subject to significant change in the future.

This approach to forecasting is purely pragmatic. The list of factors identified should be fairly short if these criteria are applied. It is important to note that factors should include those you might be able to manipulate deliberately (physicians on your staff, charges, hours of operation) as well as factors beyond your control. Forecasting rarely should be a passive process but one in which what you're interested in predicting is something on which you can have some effect.

The group involved in the factor forecasting process identifies the factors, discusses how they are likely (or how they intend them) to change in the future, and how the element you're interested in will be altered as a result. The output of such discussions rarely will be a precise estimate of the future, but rather a range of values (use rates of 800 to 850 patient days per thousand, visit rates of 3.6 to 3.8 per person). Such estimates reflect and will remind their users of the essentially guesswork nature of all forecasting and pave the way for the final step in the process: sensitivity analysis.

The idea of sensitivity analysis is to identify where in a range of values forecast for some future time a different decision would be appropriate. For example, if a forecast of 3.8 visits per year would cause you to add a physician or extender, while 3.6 would not, then your decision is sensitive to this difference. Where possible, you should strive for a more precise forecast before actually making a decision. If you can't make a better forecast, you could make a tentative decision, such as hiring a part-time or temporary physician, to wait and see rather than guess.

Where a decision is not sensitive to the range of your forecast, e.g., where you would behave the same whether use rates are 800 or 850, you can live with the range of forecasts. Sensitivity analysis tells you where you ought to use a more complex and precise forecasting method or, failing that, where you ought to make a more careful and flexible decision.

Where the factors used in your forecast approach include manipulable items, and they should, your forecast already will anticipate market objectives (Chapter 5). Where the effects of deliberate changes can be forecast and subsequently evaluated, you should be able to determine how useful and important achieving such objectives would be and how much effort and resources you could afford to spend in developing and implementing a strategy. By including in the factor forecasting group the persons who would have to implement or be affected by your strategies, you'll have paved the way for their acceptance and improved their chances of success.

DISTRIBUTING AND INTERPRETING AUDIT RESULTS

In general, the results of the market audit should be distributed widely—at least the objective returns. Your judgment as to what constitutes problem, threat, and opportunity can be withheld or reserved until after key members of the organization have examined the raw output. Considering the large number of individuals who will be affected by your findings and forecasts, a group participative approach may be useful in interpreting the results of the audit.

Facts and even forecasts that come out of the audit process may be considered legitimately as technical outputs. The identification and evaluation of problems, threats, and opportunities are largely a matter of judgment, however. Once group input and quantitative, technical inputs have been used to produce the audit results, personal, subjective value judgments are necessary in interpreting those results. Those affected by the problems, threats, and opportunities, especially those whose support and participation will be required in dealing with them, should be part of identifying and ranking exactly what they are (see Chapter 8).

In introducing the market audit for the first time, you may want to keep participation small in order to keep a low profile. If the results of the audit will lead to changes in the way a large number of persons are expected to behave, however, the low profile may be counterproductive. Given professional sensitivity to arbitrary dictation by administration, the market audit, if publicized and distributed too little, may create the feeling that professionals are being "spied on" rather than welcomed into the process. In contrast to previous patterns of starting small and expanding later, the author recommends that the audit be developed, implemented, and interpreted through wide participation within the organization.

Parts of the audit results may be distributed beyond the organization if such publication is expected to have some strategic value. Certainly boards of trustees and community advisory board members should receive copies of the results, or at least the raw output. Any attempt at secrecy is likely to fail and probably is unnecessary. Findings that may be embarrassing at first may be more useful if made known generally. It is unnecessary and often inappropriate for organizations to hide all their dirty linen. At the same time, it is by no means suggested that all or only dirty linen be aired as widely and loudly as possible. Consider the probable impact of publication on future behavior by those affected, and you'll make appropriate judgments about distribution.

SUMMARY

The market audit probably should be developed and employed incrementally in most health organizations. Natural suspicion or even antipathy regarding the appropriateness of marketing in health makes this a wise strategy. In marketing the use of marketing, it is recommended that a foot-in-the-door strategy be used, beginning with what should be the least threatening market audit possible.

The initial design of the audit content may be carried out most effectively through use of a formal group process such as Nominal Group Technique. The first phase should concentrate on the inside audit, examining existing market relationships before going on to the outside audit of potential new market relationships. Initial efforts may be fairly general, with more specific analysis reserved for areas where problems, threats, or opportunities show up in the general results. While primary focus should be on identifying and evaluating the current situation, the future or foreseeable direction in which current situations are headed also should be examined.

Forecasting techniques available for use in anticipating future problems, threats, and opportunities include three forms of trend analysis: extrapolation and simple and multiple correlation. They range from simple to complex, from mindless assumption to careful analysis. As an alternative to relying on any one of these techniques, the author suggests the use of factor forecasting. This group process technique is more flexible and subject to personal bias than quantitative alternatives, but more capable of dealing with yet-to-be experienced futures and political realities.

While the content of the market audit probably should start small and expand incrementally over time, participation in its design and implementation, plus distribution of its raw output, should be wide at the outset. Recognition of the necessity and appropriateness of using a marketing approach should be enhanced through wider involvement in designing, executing, and interpreting the market audit.

Readings

Consumer Attitudes and Behavior

Brooks, C. "Associations Among Distance, Patient Satisfaction and Utilization of Two Types of Inner-City Clinics." *Medical Care,* September/October 1973, p. 62.

Houston, C., and Pasanen, W. "Patients' Perceptions of Hospital Care." *Hospitals, JAHA* 46, 1972, p. 70.

Forst, B. "Quantifying the Patient's Preferences." in Berg, R. (ed.) *Health Status Indexes* (Chicago: Hospital Research and Educational Trust, 1973) p. 209. Paper presented at Conference on Health Status Index, Tucson, Ariz. *Health Services Research,* October 1972.

Howard, J. et al. "Humanizing Health Care—The Implications of Technology, Centralization and Self-Care." *Medical Care* 15:5, Supplement, May 1977.

Kotler, P. "From Sales Obsession to Marketing Effectiveness." *Harvard Business Review,* November/December 1977, p. 67.

Lebow, J. "Consumer Assessment of the Quality of Medical Care." *Medical Care,* 12:4, April 1974, p. 328.

Ranieri, W. "Cross-Cutting Health Priorities: A Management Trap." *Hospital and Health Services Administration* 22:4, Fall 1977, p. 24.

Steele, J. "Conceptual and Empirical Dimensions of Health Behavior." *Journal of Health and Social Behavior* 13, December 1972, p. 382.

Stratmann, W. "A Study of Consumer Attitudes About Health Care." *Medical Care* 13:7, July 1975, p. 537.

Zucherman, A. "Patient Origin Study Profiles Service Area, Evolving Patterns." *Hospital, JAHA,* July 16, 1977, p. 83.

Organizational Performance

Creditor, M.C., and V.K. "The Ecology of an Urban Voluntary Hospital: The Referral Chain." *Medical Care* 10:1, January/February 1972, p. 88.

Cunningham, "Face Fewer Admissions, Shorter Stays." *Modern Healthcare,* June 1977, p. 29.

Glick, J. "The Hospital: How Will It Survive?," *Hospital Financial Management,* January 1979, p. 12.

Hogan, S. "Your Patient Mix Affects Costs." *Hospital Financial Management,* April 1978, p. 20.

Johnson, A. "The Office Practice of Internists III: Characteristics of Patients." *JAMA* 193, 1965, p. 916.

Lovelock, C. "Concepts and Strategies for Health Marketers." *Hospital and Health Services Administration* 22:4, Fall 1977, p. 50.

"Operational Auditing Can Help Hospitals Evaluate Effectiveness, Efficiency and Economy." *Hospitals, JAHA,* March 1, 1978, p. 46.

Roberts, S. "Improving Primary Care Clinic's Effectiveness Through Assessment." *Hospitals, JAHA,* November 1, 1977, p. 123.

Roseman, C. "Problems and Prospects for Comprehensive Health Planning." *American Journal of Public Health* 62:1, January 1972, p. 16.

Ross, D., and Tripoli, F. "Fiscal Risks, Methods, Rewards Shape Community Outreach Success." *Hospitals, JAHA* 51, July 16, 1977, p. 8.

Tauber, E. "Reduce New Product Failures: Measure Needs as Well as Purchase Interest." *Journal of Marketing* 37:3, July 1973, p. 61.

Ware, J., and Boyle, B. "Physician Conduct and Other Factors That Affect Consumer Satisfaction." *Journal of Medical Education,* October 1977, p. 1036.

Part II

Utilizing Market Research

This part describes specific approaches to dealing with the realities discovered via market audits or market research. While a data base is an essential component of good marketing, it is action and results—not merely knowledge—that are the proper focus of marketing. General as well as specific responses to research findings are presented, together with examples of each based on the author's experiences in the health field. More examples of actual applications are in the cases in Part IV.

Chapter 5 discusses the formulation and use of market goals and objectives. Beginning with the kinds of data findings that arise from market research, precise definitions of goals and objectives are developed. Suggestions for formulating useful goals and objectives based on the purposes you can use them for are made. A series of applications of goals and objectives and how they relate to each other and to an overall marketing and management effort are included.

Chapter 6 examines the first three categories of organizational change that can be used as marketing strategies. These are, first, changes in product—the positive benefits markets derive from doing business with you. Second are place factors, arrangements, and mechanisms whereby markets avail themselves of your product. Third are price factors, the negative flip side of the advantages your product offers: the costs to your markets of doing business and, specifically, of doing it with you.

Chapter 7 focuses on the fourth strategic category: promotion. By definition, this includes everything you say and all mechanisms you use to communicate to your markets about product, place, and price. It describes the effects you seek in promotional efforts, how to focus efforts appropriately, and both medium and message considerations you should employ. It presents practical examples of promotional efforts that have been used by health care organizations, although a more detailed example is presented in a case in Chapter 16.

Chapter 8 describes a widely useful management challenge: the determination of preference or priority. It discusses a variety of applications of priority setting, including a number of different definitions of what the results mean. Specific techniques for determining the best, most important, worst, or otherwise superlative choice are described. The use of priority setting in ranking problems, threats, opportunities and alternative actions and in evaluating results is covered.

Chapter 5

Market Goals and Objectives

Thousands of words have been written about goals and objectives in general. This has not resulted in any unanimity of opinion about what they are, how they relate to each other, how they are used, or how to formulate effective versions. For purposes of this book, precise definitions of both goals and objectives are used and the reasons for these definitions explained. The purposes and uses of goals and objectives are discussed, as well as how they interact with each other, with the audit process, and with strategy development.

PURPOSE

The first point to recognize is that market goals and objectives are meant to achieve some purpose, to do you some good. Rather than merely accept the necessity of having goals and objectives, it would be better to start by identifying what you want them to do for you. Expressions of your targets, the ends you strive toward, should:

- clarify to yourself and to others why you're in business
- justify your continued existence and growth
- motivate your employees and supporters to work harder
- focus your planning and action efforts toward specific expected outcomes
- monitor your progress and evaluate your contribution

How good your goals and objectives are will be determined by how well they perform one or more of these functions. This discussion is geared to identifying the types of goals and objectives and relations between and among them, and proposing methods for formulating and employing them that will optimize the contribution they make to your marketing efforts.

DEFINITION

Market goals and objectives should be defined as follows:

Goal: a future state of an impact, behavior, causal factor, environment, or competition situation you'd like to be in someday and plan to expend effort toward

Objective: a future state of impact, behavior, causal factors, environment, or competition you are determined to accomplish by a specific time

Both are descriptions of something you want to be true in the future. An objective carries with it your determination to achieve a specific achievement by a specific time while a goal promises a general obligation to achieve it eventually. Your statements of desired futures shouldn't be casual wishes but commitments toward general (goals) or specific (objectives) efforts to achieve a future that otherwise wouldn't occur. Foreseeable futures that will occur without your intervention are forecasts, not targets. It is the commitment to intervention for the purpose of achieving change that makes a goal or an objective.

GOALS

Goals themselves tend to be lofty and vague in many cases. They may seek to:

- meet the health needs of the community
- ensure a healthful environment
- ensure equitable access to quality health care at reasonable costs.

Such lofty rhetoric may serve some of the purposes of goals but fail in others. They make focus of effort, motivation, and evaluation very difficult, though they may justify your existence and attract support. To get the full use out of such goals, each would have to be defined specifically and probably expressed more clearly, such as to:

- provide all medical services needed and expected to be used by the residents of Anywhere, U.S.A.
- eliminate all health hazards from the environment in Anywhere

- ensure that all people can get the health care they require, of quality and cost acceptable to them and to providers and payers

Such global goals, however, are so vast as to represent more policy or mission statements than precise descriptions of future outcomes. The best, most useful goals are those without action verbs describing what you will do, (ensure, provide, improve, etc.) but that precisely indicate a new situation within an organization (your psychographics, demographics, behavior, and impacts) or outside it (their psychographics, demographics, impacts, the environment, and competition). These more precise goals should both define and make explicit what you intend to accomplish and, when added together, constitute the fulfillment of your mission.

Goals should be related to each other in meaningful ways. Ultimately the reason for and worth of all your goals should be determined by impacts: the health of your organization and of the community you serve. The reasons for achieving changes in any of the other factors should relate clearly to the impacts such changes will have on why you're ultimately in business. Goals that don't relate clearly to expected and desired impacts should be reconsidered thoroughly. The number of goals of an organization should be fairly small, under 20 and preferably fewer than 10, or the prospects of achieving the goals themselves and the purposes for having them will be compromised.

OBJECTIVES

Each objective should be a partial accomplishment of a goal, a phase through which you *must* pass on the way to the goal itself. It is a description of a future state of affairs, but one you have a firm commitment to achieve by a stated time. If your goals are vague and general, at least your objectives should be clear and specific. Objectives are designed more to focus effort, motivate performance, and monitor accomplishments than to achieve any external or rhetorical purpose, although they may help in these latter efforts as well.

An objective is a promise you make to yourself and anyone to whom you distribute descriptions of objectives. Each should be chosen carefully since promises should be made only where you are confident they can and will be kept. Some unforeseeable events very well may prevent or delay the achievement of some objectives but these should be rare events. The reporting of excuses rather than accomplishment should be the exception rather than the rule.

In order to accomplish the purpose of the title of this book, *Marketing by Objectives,* it is essential that objectives be considered carefully and thoroughly. Like goals, each should be justified ultimately in terms of actual or expected impacts on your or the community's health. You may not always be able to tie a change in behavior, psychographics, demographics, environment, or competition to a specific impact in practice, but you should be able to build a confident logical linkage in your analysis.

Objectives may relate to goals in a number of ways. In cases where a goal is vague or general, the objective in effect may define it for you. Thus, if your goal relates to improving the timeliness of your service, an objective might be that by next year 90 percent of all patients should be seen within 60 seconds of arrival. Each year, instead of improving this measure, you may adopt other objectives, reflecting different indicators of timeliness or addressing other services. The objectives are narrow measures of a more general concern. The presumption would be that when you run out of measures to improve, you've accomplished your goal.

Objectives also may be a category of a goal. Should your goal be to eradicate all preventable, communicable diseases in a community, an objective might be to eradicate rubella. Similarly, an objective could be a segment of a goal, such as to eradicate all communicable diseases in a specific zip code or census tract. Both would qualify as objectives since they must be achieved or passed through in order to accomplish the goal. Each also could serve as a subgoal, if a specific time frame is not included.

The one step to avoid in developing objectives out of goals is to choose an objective that has only an incidental or perhaps ill-defined relationship to a goal. This happens most often when an objective is a statement of how you intend to achieve a goal (i.e., a strategy) rather than an intermediate benchmark on the way to accomplishing that goal. Whenever an objective describes what you intend to do (activity) rather than the outcome it is expected to have (accomplishment), you probably are talking strategy. While strategies are necessary, they are to be chosen after an objective is suggested and more than one alternative strategy is examined. The danger of stating a strategy as an objective is that it actually may not be an effective, or the most effective or efficient, mechanism for achieving your goal.

If your goal is to achieve 90 percent occupancy in a hospital, and your objective is stated in terms of recruiting additional medical staff, you're skipping a few logical steps. The most obvious objectives would be to achieve 80 percent occupancy by next year, 85 percent in two years, etc. By stating your objective in terms of a specific strategy (recruiting physicians) you ignore some obvious alternative choices:

- reducing your bed complement
- getting larger market shares from current medical staff

- expanding emergency room or ambulatory care programs
- increasing satisfaction of patients

The same kind of warning applies to selecting objectives or goals in the first place. Any goal or objective stated in terms of behavior, causal factors, environment, or competition should be justified in terms of its anticipated impact. Thus, an objective focused on changing behavior (yours or your market's) should be expected to produce or protect an important measure of impact: your health or that of your service community.

Any objective relative to a goal, or any goal itself, should be examined by asking the question: is that situation self-evidently superior to the current situation in and of itself or because of what we assume it means or affects? For example, are higher occupancy or more services clearly better per se, or only because of what they mean to your financial health? If it is their instrumental rather than intrinsic value that makes them desirable, you should be sure that at least they are the best instrument, the best indicator of your real interest. The most disappointing goals and objectives are those that don't mean anything important even when they're accomplished.

FORMULATING GOALS AND OBJECTIVES

To get the most out of your market goals and objectives, you should formulate them with appropriate care. In drafting them, you should consider both technical and political realities and consequences. Each will be discussed in detail, together with some of the potential consequences of ignoring either.

Technical Requirements

The first requirement in formulating goals and objectives is that each be developed relative to a known present situation. It may be easier to identify what you'd like to be the case in the abstract without bothering to find out what is now the case, but it isn't very useful. Especially is this true for objectives, since you should commit yourself only to achieving changes you are confident you can accomplish. Without knowing where you are now, and how much change would be required to achieve the objective, you can't make an intelligent commitment.

Second, the goals and objectives you formulate should represent better situations than you would anticipate to result from "business as usual." Goals and objectives are meant to focus and justify new or increased effort rather than be the expected result of current activities. The market audit, or any service-specific planning and research effort, should forecast what the future promises as the expected result of what you're doing now. Any goal or objective should portray a better future than that and should be used to formulate a new strategy. Where the future expected to result from continuing current efforts is optimal or at least acceptable, no goals or objectives should be necessary.

While goals are descriptions of what you'd like your market situation to be eventually, they should be reasonable expectations rather than risk the frustration of your never seeming to make much progress in their direction. Goals may be stated even in terms of direction rather than an endpoint to avoid such frustration. Thus, goal statements may be made in terms of "as low as possible" or "optimal" levels of a situation, rather than precise quantitative terms. Objectives then can be used to identify specific achievable benchmarks in the direction of your goal.

Objectives always should be drafted in pencil on erasable paper at first. Since each represents a commitment to achievement, it should be adopted permanently only after you are sure it can and will be accomplished. Thus, once a draft version of an objective is formulated, alternative strategies should be examined, the feasibility of their implementation and probability of success analyzed, and a commitment made to implement one. Based on the expected outcome of the strategy, and the confident belief that the required resources, support, or permission can be obtained to implement it, a final version of the objective can be adopted.

The draft version of the objective serves to focus and motivate discussion and analysis of strategies, implementation, feasibility, and results. Only after and as a result of such discussions should the final version of the objective be approved. This final statement of the objective then will serve as the basis for motivating and focusing actual effort toward achievement. The accomplishment of objectives then serves to motivate further progress toward the goal.

To employ a marketing perspective, the focus of marketing objectives must be on behavior. It is the understanding of what motivates marketplace behavior that represents marketing's unique contribution to the planning and development of health services. Any goals or objectives related to psychographics, demographics, environment, or competition should be formulated and evaluated in terms of their expected effects on behavior. The market goals and objectives that specifically address changes in behavior should be formulated and evaluated then in terms of their expected impact on organizational and community health.

Political Requirements

In addition to the technical requirements and pitfalls in formulating market goals and objectives, there are important political realities as well. Since objectives are immediate and goals are long-term commitments by the organization, a number of persons are likely to be affected by them. Those affected may include those who, for the changes you propose, must:

- approve (board of trustees, regulatory agencies, governmental commissions)
- support (donors, third party payment organizations)
- participate in (physicians, professional and nonprofessional employees)
- be affected by (patients, the community at large)

Individuals whose support for changes you may need, or whose opposition to such changes you'd rather avoid, should be identified early. In most cases, you should have done so as part of the market audit process. If not, or if you are developing specific goals and objectives that are not direct results of a comprehensive market audit, you certainly should identify important constituents as part of setting goals and objectives.

How many such persons to involve, when in the process to bring them in, and how to accommodate them are matters of judgment and management style rather than market recipes. For ad hoc program- or problem-specific goals and objectives, a task force rather than standing committee approach would be more realistic. Where an overall, organizationwide set of goals and objectives is being formulated out of market audit results, a permanent committee would be more useful. The more persons you bring in early, the less control you retain over the results of their deliberations. The fewer individuals, or the later you involve them, the greater the risk that they may object to the decisions reached and fail to provide the support needed.

External organizations whose regulatory approval (e.g., certificate of need) or financial support (government grant, foundation) you require may not be able to serve on a task force or committee discussing your market goals and objectives. You still may use a political marketing approach to some advantage, however. Marketing is based on exchange theory: the notion that people will change the way they behave if they get something for it in return.

While this theory may seem to suggest bribing members of external organizations whose support you wish, that is by no means the only choice and certainly not a recommended one. The essence of marketing is identifying what kinds of benefits or positive changes in their situation others are interested in, then seeing which ones you can produce to mutual advantage. By identifying and understanding what motivates such organizations, you can determine what advantages your goals and objectives might create for them.

Ideally, individual health care organizations, the communities they serve, and the planning or regulatory agencies that supervise that service should have substantial interests and motivation in common. Some differences of opinion, priorities, or assumptions probably are inevitable but they need not be the sole basis for interaction. By concentrating on interests all have in common, the health care organization can identify how its proposed changes (expressed in goals, objectives, strategies) will benefit all. By understanding what those interests and potential benefits are, the organization can formulate the kinds of goals, objectives, and strategies that will have the greatest mutual benefits.

Within the organization, important power figures—both formal and informal leaders—should be identified. Their interests and the extent to which they would be affected by proposed changes should be examined. One way of accomplishing this is through careful technical analysis. Another is through their participation, representing their own interests, in discussions of such proposed changes. At a minimum, leaders among the medical staff, employees, and the governing/advisory board should be included in analysis or discussions. Other representatives of the patient market and community may be useful in preparing for approval, support, acceptance, or use of service changes proposed.

APPLICATIONS

The purposes of goals and objectives are obvious examples of the general applications for which they may be used. These will be discussed in some detail, together with some uses of goals and objectives that may apply to specific cases. Both the general and specific applications should be considered in formulating such statements in the first place.

Clarification of purpose, role, and mission is one application of goals and objectives. By formulating goals and objectives in terms of precise and measurable changes in reality, you can clarify your reason for being in business to your own people (medical staff, employees, boards) as well as to your publics (patients, supports, regulators, competition, and community). Where your role and mission statements may be vague and general, your goals and objectives should be more precise and specific. To achieve such clarification, you should formulate goals to be understood by the external publics to which you communicate them.

Justification of your continued existence and long-term growth, presumably desired by all organizations, may be assisted through effective formulation and publication of your goals and objectives. Most useful in this regard will be those describing external impacts, statements of community health, satisfaction, and benefit. Specific compilations of your goals and objectives in this area, together perhaps with your plans for your own behavior, would be appropriate for external publication. This should help you achieve necessary support, approvals, and acceptance by external publics.

Motivation of members of your organization should be furthered by appropriate use of your goals and objectives. Understanding and recognition of their role in achieving such targets should clarify the worth of their efforts to each employee, medical staff member, or volunteer. Periodic achievement of and reward for accomplishing specific objectives should reinforce the general motivational values of goals and objectives. The objectives you employ in this effort must be both achievable and important enough, as well as of sufficient short-term nature and continuing progress, to serve this function. All persons you wish to help motivate through objectives must be able to see their specific contribution to them and notice progress in the appropriate direction, as well as enjoy the commensurate rewards.

Goals and objectives should serve to focus both planning and action toward their achievement. Goals should be formulated in the confident expectation that some way will be found to achieve them. Therefore, some notion as to the availability and feasibility of action toward their accomplishment should be in mind when they are discussed. Objectives, particularly, should be developed through careful examination of specific strategies and with a commitment to both their implementation and success. Knowledge of the outcome of actions should maintain their direction as well as intensity.

Monitoring and evaluating the effectiveness of your marketing program certainly is one of the most important values and applications of goals and objectives. Each objective—whether it covers impacts, behavior, causal factors, external, or competitive situations—should be capable of checking to note progress. How valuable progress toward each is should be examined as part of developing objectives and strategies. How much progress actually is achieved should be monitored to evaluate strategies, reward effort, and motivate future activity. Strategies that don't work should be analyzed to identify flaws in the market analysis that decided on them. Strategies that do work should be examined anyway to discover whether they did so because or in spite of market analysis that led to their adoption. Only if both the analysis and the strategy worked should they be repeated.

On top of these general applications appropriate for any goal or objective formulation effort, specific applications also are possible. In some cases, publication of general or specific program intentions (new services, new markets) may dissuade competitive organizations from considering their own possibilities in the area. The reverse also may happen in some instances and your intentions actually stimulate their competitive development. You must use your own judgment as to the appropriateness and probable effects of this application in practice.

Another possible application would be to recruit specific participants in a market effort. By developing goals and objectives related to a new or expanded program, you may be able to convince medical or other health professionals to join your organization. You must be careful, of course, to make sure such goals and objectives (and hence the reasons for recruiting new staff) can be achieved. Potential barriers, in terms of financial requirements, regulatory approvals, etc., should be anticipated and preparations made for them. Marketing, like politics, is the art of the possible, but it also should be the art of the probable.

Still a third specific application might be to obtain preaction approval for specific program plans. In many areas, local planning agencies automatically grant certificate-of-need approval to applications that are consistent with your overall plan, provided your plan has been approved. The specific program objectives—how you intend to behave if approved—should simplify the review process and prevent expenditure of effort toward program changes that won't be approved.

SUMMARY

The starting point in formulating goals and objectives is to identify the purposes you wish them to serve. A goal is defined as a state you'd like to achieve in the future, and intend to strive toward. An objective is a state you are determined to accomplish by a specific date. Both goals and objectives should be justified and evaluated in terms of their impacts on the organization's and the community's health, broadly defined. Objectives are intermediate stages through which you must pass on the way to a goal. They may serve to clarify or segment a goal, but should not be strategies you intend to employ to achieve one.

To get the most out of your goals and objectives, you should be sure:

- that you start from a description of the current market situation
- that they be reasonable and foreseeable results of implementable action
- that objectives are formulated in draft form and adopted finally only when you feel confident in their accomplishment
- that objectives focus on behavior changes that will occur if other changes are achieved and that are themselves justified by the impacts expected

To attain the maximum acceptance and achievement of your goals and objectives, you should incorporate analysis or participation of persons and organizations whose support is essential or whose opposition could be detrimental to their realization. Market concepts and techniques can be used to identify and respond to their interests and ensure that your goals and objectives represent significant mutual benefit.

Goals and objectives should serve to clarify your organization's mission and role, justify its existence and growth, motivate and reward effort, focus planning and action, and help you monitor and evaluate progress. In addition, in specific instances they may help you discourage competition, recruit professionals, or enlist regulatory approvals. To accomplish each purpose most effectively, the formulation, description, and publication of goals and objectives must be tailored accordingly.

Chapter 6

Market Strategies

Having specified your marketing goals and objectives, based on your understanding of how and why individuals and organizations behave, you next plan how to achieve your objectives through your market strategies. Since marketing is based on exchange theory, it assumes that whenever you seek to alter the behavior of markets with respect to your organization, you must alter your organization's behavior with respect to them. This chapter discusses the types of changes you might make in your organization in order to promote changes in the behavior of the markets that have been targeted in your goals and objectives.

There are four categories of changes you can make in the way your organization behaves in order to alter or protect behavior by your markets—the four classic *Ps* of marketing:

Product: the benefits or positive results that markets derive out of doing business with you, using the services you offer in the way you offer them

Place: the hours, location, eligibility rules, referrals, or admission arrangements that make it possible, easy, or difficult for markets to use your product

Price: the costs or negative side effects markets must bear in order to do business with you, using the services you offer the way you offer them

Promotion: what and how you inform markets about your product, place, and price (see Chapter 7)

PRODUCT

The essence of dealing with your *product*, the benefits people or organizations derive from entering into a market relationship with you, is that such benefits must be viewed from *their* perspective. How do they anticipate becoming better off and well-served, and how do they actually become so, through doing business with you? In examining patient behavior, what advantages do they derive from their use of health services: relief from pain, elimination of disability, alleviation of anxiety, the promise of improved functioning? You must be able to view their expected and realized benefits from their perspective in order to understand their satisfaction and to predict and influence their behavior.

Surveys of markets are likely to be the only way you can learn what the public derives from using health services but, fortunately, such surveys have been done by others. These suggest the kinds of "product" attributes in which people are most interested.

By examining how people view your current products through your market audit, and through understanding the attributes that most strongly affect consumer choice, you can design new services or modifications to existing programs accordingly. Through understanding how your products are viewed by their current and prospective users, especially where their choice is an important factor in their use behavior, you can better develop service responses that meet their expectations. Since your purpose must be to develop services that will be used appropriately and efficiently, the ability to design and implement service programs that will attract sufficient use is critical.

In recruiting physicians, the challenge is identical: to identify attributes of community location and hospital staff membership that are most important to physician choice and to use such knowledge to predict and influence physician decisions. Unless community characteristics can be manipulated, which is difficult in most cases, you will use your knowledge of which factors affect choice to identify higher probability physician segments. A rural hospital would be better off focusing its recruiting efforts on physicians who were born and raised in rural areas, or whose spouses were.

For attributes of the hospital (size, age of physical plant, range of services offered) some will also be fixed, and not subject to your manipulation. In such cases, you should identify which of your fixed characteristics would appeal to whom and focus your recruiting efforts on the appropriate segments. Primary physicians, young physicians, or older ones whose children are grown and who are tired of the pace of urban life all may be target segments for rural hospitals with basic services. You must be able to view what you offer from the perspective of the physicians you're trying to recruit in order to predict who would be likely to make what decisions.

Many attributes of the hospital and community can be manipulated, however. By identifying what factors motivate physician choice, you can enhance your offering accordingly and increase your success rates in recruitment. Prospects of financial rewards can be augmented or simply guaranteed through contracts, start-up subsidies, etc. Some of the costs of setting up practice can be absorbed by the hospital: rental of space, employment of office help, recordkeeping, billing, etc. Doctors' office buildings have been overused in many urban communities as a recruitment device but still may be useful in suburban and rural areas.

The small elements about a choice of where to practice and admit or refer patients may be as important as the larger factors. Quality and timing of communications, parking privileges, physicians' lounge areas, and activities for spouses during a recruitment visit may be telling concerns. Human motivation is complex, and relatively minor amenities may be the most important factors among alternatives facing the physician. What you consider minor may well be considered major by the individuals whose decisions you're hoping to influence.

There is no guaranteed successful method for recruiting physicians, of course. The sheer growth in their numbers and slight shifts toward more family and primary care practitioners may well ease the recruitment problems in some areas, but you still probably would want to recruit the best as well as the right number of physicians. Through examining what you do or could offer to physicians from their perspective, and understanding their motivation, you should be able to enhance your offering and improve your success.

The care and feeding of current physicians admitting or referring patients, or of other referral organizations, also is important. You must be sure that what you offer to prospective recruits doesn't upset your current physician or agency market. Including them in your discussion of recruitment strategies may be one way to ensure their feelings won't be hurt, but it also may constrain severely what strategies you can use. Care must be taken to point out to existing staff and to referral agencies the advantages to *them* of adding to your market. Here again, understanding what motivates them will help you identify what kinds of advantages would be worth emphasizing.

New primary care physicians should augment referrals to specialists and take workload pressures off the current supply of family practitioners. Additional and especially new kinds of specialists will enable more patients to be treated locally and reduce the number who are "lost" to distant referral centers. Adding to laboratory and x-ray use will help the entire hospital financially. Such advantages should be cited only if they truly will occur, however. It is always bad marketing to mislead the consumer, especially if repeated use or loyal relationships are desired.

PLACE

The extent to which your products are readily available, convenient to use, etc., is a sufficiently important attribute of your product to warrant separate attention. Like product, the positive and negative aspects of your *place* must be viewed from the perspective of the market, rather than from yours. At a minimum, place considerations from your patients' perspective include such factors as:

- your days and hours of operation, relative to the days and hours your markets find time available to use your services
- your location, relative to the modes of transportation available to your markets and their current and preferred travel patterns
- your parking arrangements, such as distance from your service site and the cost and difficulty of finding space
- your eligibility criteria, admissions or registration procedures, and reception process
- your waiting time to obtain an appointment, to be first seen, and total time required to receive an episode of care

Hours

Originally, private physicians and public clinics incorporated hours convenient to the working public. As technical dependence and organized health care increased, the dominant mode came to be offering services during the normal working day and week. For markets that have difficulty or that pay a price in lost wages for using services during the normal working day, this represents a hardship. By identifying when individuals can use services most easily, you can enhance their likelihood of doing so.

Compromises are likely to be necessary here. In a seller's market, consumers have to live with what the provider does. If you can't convince your medical staff or employees to offer services at other than normal working hours, you're stuck. The risk is always that a competitor might succeed where you fail and thus attract a substantial share of your market before you belatedly react. By knowing the extent of your market's preference for better hours and estimating the probability of your competition's being able to offer better hours, you could preact rather than react to such a challenge.

Location

Where you are located most often is not open to manipulation, save once. Facilities for most health services are hard to move. Some options do exist, however, through mobile clinics, renting space, etc. A classic example exists in the Soviet Union on the Moscow–Vladivostok railway where a traveling clinic delivers care to the small communities along the right-of-way. Trial locations can be used via mobile trailers or rented space until the most acceptable and successful one is identified.

Parking

The bane of most health care programs seems to be parking. Physicians, employees, patients, and visitors have to be accommodated at hospitals and it never seems possible to do so adequately. Offering a shuttle bus from a remote site may be useful where space constraints prohibit adequate onsite space, though parking high rises are another option. Both the safety and convenience of parking are a major concern, as many core-city hospitals have found to their chagrin.

Eligibility

What the prospective patient *views* as your intended as well as eligible market is more important than what is true. People who do not feel welcome are likely to be put off as much as those who are categorically eligible. Where misunderstandings exist, clear and constant communication is about your only remedy—unless you wish to serve specifically only those who view themselves as welcome. Your eligibility rules and communications should be such that individuals can determine readily in advance whether they will be welcomed. Those who would be welcomed but don't come and those who aren't eligible but do come are both failures of your communications.

Waiting Time

Along with parking, waiting time is the most common annoyance in health care. Delays in getting appointments, in being seen upon arrival at your site, in being processed through a series of services are separate and equally negative aspects of your place. Some waiting time is inevitable if you wish to optimize productivity of your expensive resources. Much could be avoided through better prediction of the level and variability of demand for your services, combined with a desire to minimize waiting time and improve patient flows. Some specific suggestions on this are discussed in Chapter 10.

Waiting time often is used to ration the use of services the organization delivers reluctantly. This has been a common practice among hospitals for decades. It would be wise for such institutions to consider first their reluctance regarding ambulatory care. It is likely that, in the future, the overall financial health and contribution of hospitals will depend more and more on ambulatory services.[1] Where this is true, the deliberate or inadvertant incon-

---

[1] D. Wendt, "The Hospital As Medical Practitioner," *Hospitals, JAHA,* December 1, 1978, p. 41.

venience to patients of waiting will reduce the potential for optimal or even adequate market shares, wherever a competitor is willing to offer a better deal.

To the extent that any of your place attributes facilitate or hinder your market relationships, they should be incorporated in design and modification of service programs. In a noncompetitive situation, inconveniences of place may be accepted by your markets as unavoidable. They may even be welcomed as part of the notion that if it doesn't taste bad, the medicine can't be effective. Busy waiting rooms and long waits for an appointment testify to the popularity and presumably to the quality of a provider. There's always the risk, however, that a competitor will come along and offer greater convenience, attracting away a substantial market share.

A classic example of the waiting time effect has occurred among a number of newly developed Health Maintenance Organizations. When first opened, the HMOs have lots of room, plenty of staff, and few patients as enrollment starts slowly. This makes it easy for patients to get appointments and means they rarely will have to wait long in the waiting room. As enrollment increases, however, a more normal waiting time for both appointments and contact develops, and old patients feel quality has gone down. This reality suggests HMOs might be wise to control waiting time artificially to the level they anticipate will be normal, rather than to promote dissatisfaction by having to go from good to worse.

PRICE

Price considerations are especially complex in health care. The health care marketplace is abnormal with respect to price in that such a small portion actually is paid by the consumer at the time of use. Moreover, the main actor in determining what, when, and which services will be used is the physician, who doesn't pay the cost and, in fact, benefits financially from providing services. Such a market situation is not replicated in any other industry.

In effect, there are two categories of price in health care—(1) the direct and indirect out-of-pocket costs to the consumer for using services, and (2) all other negative aspects of the use of a specific service from a specific provider. The extent to which one category or the other plays a more or less important part in decisions about use should determine how your organization deals with price issues. Most of the common approaches to pricing by health care organizations are inappropriate from a marketing perspective.

There are two reasons for being concerned about price, both out-of-pocket and other. First, unless the market views the positive benefits you provide (product) under the circumstances you offer them (place) worth the negative costs they entail (price), that market will not use the product. It would not represent a fair bargain to users and wouldn't be worth it. Second, unless the product/price or benefit/cost relationship you offer is at least as good as, and you hope better than, what is offered by competitors, the market will not turn to you for the product. Why should it?

Out-of-Pocket Prices

The amount a consumer has to pay, either at the time of use or to the provider of services as a direct and specific result of that use, is the direct out-of-pocket cost of care. The indirect out-of-pocket costs include whatever losses in wages, transportation, parking, baby-sitting, or other expenditures are required for a patient to use your services. Both have to be examined from the perspective of the market and in the context of the competition. Some out-of-pocket costs are easy to measure (direct) but others will require surveys such as the market audit to identify (indirect). It isn't just the costs that concern you, however, but the attitude of the market toward them.

Traditional pricing practices among health care organizations address only direct price. As such, they fall short of understanding, predicting, and influencing market behavior very effectively. Even in making direct price decisions (charges), however, health care organizations typically fail to use a market perspective. The most common approach to charges is cost-based. This, in effect, is basing your charges on what someone else charges you, independent of what your customers expect or are willing to pay. Such an approach may seem logical in an abstract sense but may be counterproductive in terms of your markets. Some services, especially where the patient has little choice, are likely to have demand that is not elastic to price. Charges higher or lower than what you charge would have little effect on demand.

Other services, however, may be very elastic as to price. Those where the consumer has a choice as to whether to use care, which type of care to use (e.g., long-term institution vs. home care) or where to obtain it are likely to have demands that do vary, depending on out-of-pocket charges. If you analyze the marginal expenditure/revenue expected for different charge levels, you might well discover your organization would be better off with higher or lower charges. Since much health care is reimbursed for costs, of course, this analysis should be done only where your income is at least significantly affected by charges. This may occur even where patients don't pay much of out-of-pocket charges themselves but where deductibles or coinsurance give them some stake in limiting their use of services.

Another approach to pricing common to ambulatory health care is the what-the-market-will-bear approach. This is reflected in finding out what competitors charge and pegging your own prices accordingly. While on the surface a market-pricing approach, this fails to take into account full costs or attitudes by markets regarding charges. In many cases it may be that individuals would pay more for the services you offer because of your presumed higher quality. In other circumstances, only a price lower than the competition would attract customers away from their established patterns. Where the indirect out-of-pocket costs give you an advantage or disadvantage over the competition, you waste that advantage or suffer the disadvantage unwittingly unless you incorporate them in your pricing decisions.

Unless you know what patients experience in both direct and indirect, out-of-pocket costs, taking into account how much they'll actually pay, you can't set maximum benefit from your pricing decisions. Unless you further examine the specific effects of less use on your finances and mission that might result from higher charges, or more use from lower charges, you can't claim to be using marketing analysis to its greatest effect. It is the product/price relationship you must consider, rather than the price alone. Your consideration must focus on how pricing will affect consumers as well as how it would affect you.

Other Costs

Where out-of-pocket charges have little effect, or even when they do, other costs are likely to enter into market decisions on health care. Most health services are likely to involve some pain or discomfort, anxiety, or indignities. As with other aspects of price, such costs must be viewed from the perspective of the consumer, even when they verge into psychological, social, or spiritual effects. What makes consideration of other costs more difficult is that:

- *their* costs usually don't produce any benefits to your organization
- their costs are very difficult to measure and compare to benefits
- your attempts to do something about their costs will cost you something, and the prospect of benefit to you is likely to be indistinct

The category of *other costs* includes items that are the direct or indirect result of your behavior. Many are related closely to your place behavior: the indignity and anxiety of long waits, and the danger of parking in or walking to the area of your location (fear of mugging or rape). Others may result from your desire for efficient high quality service: patients feeling rushed, treated as cases or diseases rather than as people, backless and shapeless gowns for inpatients, inconvenient hours for meals, etc. Still others are side effects of what you do: nosocomial infections or iatrogenic conditions.

As pressures to hold down costs of health care mount, they are likely to be felt most severely in areas that are considered amenities, important to patients but not to health professionals. Reducing amenities may have far greater detrimental effects on behavior and more serious effects on the organization's and the community's health, however, than cost reductions in some more essential area (e.g., administration, equipment). Changes in services designed to reduce costs should be made in anticipation of their full effects on the organization and the community, not merely the obvious reductions in cost.

PHYSICIANS/REFERRAL AGENCIES

Previous discussion of price has focused on the cost to consumers of health services. Equally important are price considerations to physicians and agencies who admit or refer patients. The price to them, from their perspective, must be validated by the benefits they derive from doing business with you. Since direct out-of-pocket costs rarely are a concern, this discussion of costs to your "agents" will focus on indirect and other costs.

For physicians, the chief indirect costs are likely to be time lost from practice. Any professional whose income depends on how much time is available to see patients is likely to be extremely sensitive to time demands. Requirements for serving on committees, attending board meetings, completing medical records, etc., will be viewed by physicians as costs of doing business with you, whether or not you derive benefit from them.

Many of these costs are necessary because of quality of care concerns, licensing or accreditation requirements, etc. Recognizing how physicians view such requirements, however, you should be sure that meetings, record-keeping, etc. are kept minimally complex, time consuming, and onerous. It is easy to be self-righteous about what physicians must do in the interests of quality as their professional obligation, etc., but if you lose medical staff, both you and the community will suffer for righteousness's sake.

Referring physicians and agencies are a special problem. Their greatest cost is likely to be their loss of contact with "their" patient, or fear of the permanent loss of that patient. This is especially common among local physicians referring to a distant medical center, but equally a problem for a single or narrow-service agency referring to a multiservice organization such as a hospital.

The natural competitive advantages of the university medical center, specialist, or full-service hospital compared to the local general hospital, family practitioner, or single-function agency are well known. It is almost a tradition in health care for the "superior" organizations to belittle or ignore the local provider, despite the negative market effects this has. The loss of face or feared loss of patients that tend to accompany upward referrals will tend to keep them at a minimum, even where fear of malpractice or other concerns tend to promote greater referrals.

By making medical staff and employees aware of these costs, the referral recipient can hope to reduce the belittling or patient pirating. Even where the recipient does provide a truly superior product, it is by no means necessary to engage in comparative advertising, and its ethics are debatable. Of course, all this must be tempered by concern that patients should continue to receive quality of care, and if the referring agency really is dangerous to the patient, marketing realities may appropriately give way to professional ethics.

As in all marketing decisions, the costs vs. the benefits of altering your organization's pricing decisions regarding physicians and referral agencies should be examined in full. Altering your price to them may affect your product, price, or place. Special provisions made for a few physicians or agencies to attract or retain them may anger providers who are even more important to you. Through a comprehensive market audit, you should have the information base necessary to evaluate and make effective pricing decisions.

SUMMARY

There are four principal categories of changes your organization can make in itself, of which three (product, place, and price) are discussed in this chapter. Product refers to the positive consequences people derive from market relations with you. Place covers the hours of initiating and maintaining such relations. Price includes all negative consequences of using your product, only one part of which is out-of-pocket payments.

Product considerations involve how people benefit, as they view it, from doing business with you. They include how patients gain (cure, stress reduction, increased mobility, protection) and how physicians benefit (equipment, trained staff, information, colleagues). The specific preferences by market segments for different product attributes should be identified through market research and used in designing programs, selecting markets, or developing promotions. You must design and implement benefits that attract individuals to your place in recognition of your price. Place considerations include all those factors that determine how easy or difficult it is to use your product. Where positive, place considerations enhance your product; where difficult, place factors increase your price. Which way they act, to what extent, and for whom should be considered in making program decisions on hours, location, parking, eligibility criteria, and waiting time. Place factors, like product and price, should be manipulated to optimize your market relations. To do so requires that you be able to understand such factors from the perspective of your markets.

Price factors include out-of-pocket expenditures, both direct and indirect, required of markets that do business with you. They also include other negative consequences, including loss of time, of dignity, pain, discomfort, anxiety, and nosocomial and iatrogenic conditions. Like product and place, the effects of price factors on market decisions can be understood only if they are viewed from the perspective of those who pay them. The price you require people to pay must be outweighed by the benefits you promise and deliver or people won't use the product. Your offer of product vs. price must compete effectively against other available alternatives.

Chapter 7

Promotional Strategies

The word "promotion" unfortunately has more negative than positive connotations and inadequately describes the fourth factor subject to change in order to alter market relationships. On the other hand, it probably is the one common notion in what most people think of as marketing—a focus on advertising and sales. It was deliberately left for last in this discussion because it truly follows after and is last in importance compared to product, price, and place. On the other hand, it is given a full chapter because of the great interest it generates and the wide array of possibilities for its use.

The essence of promotion is communication. It specifically does not mean "packaging" or hucksterism, as in free giveaways, parades, or trading stamps, although these may serve a communications function. The classic example of promotion in health care probably is the "bonus" giveaway used by Sunrise Hospital in Las Vegas: a drawing for a free two-week "recuperative" cruise to those admitted to the hospital on Friday or Saturday.[1] While advertising of the offer was an important part of the strategy, its essence was product enhancement, giving people something more if they behaved differently.

This particular example already had passed through a price-changing strategy that had failed. Sunrise had offered a 5 percent discount to persons admitted on Friday or Saturday, but since health insurance covered most costs, this proposal didn't change patient behavior. The product enhancement did work, resulting in a 30 percent increase in weekend occupancy. Such a result probably wouldn't have been achieved without promotion, the communication of the offer to an interested public. However, it was the product change that presumably altered behavior, not simply a change in communication.

By definition, promotion refers only to communication of information to potential and actual markets. It is designed to make markets aware of, inter-

---

[1] C. Marshall, "Ethical Aspects of Advertising Debated," *Modern Healthcare* 7:4, April 1977, p. 48.

ested in, desirous of, committed to, and finally a customer of, your products. This hierarchy of effects is about as much as can be asked of communications. Further commitment by your markets to repeated, even regular, use of your product, or to serving as a promoter of your product to acquaintances and colleagues, is presumed to result only from their actual experience with your product, place, and price.

Even within this narrow definition of promotion, however, there are numerous possibilities for attracting new markets or changing market behavior. A whole field of health promotion has grown up, with communication the chief technique, through what is called health education. While our success in changing behavior through pure education (communication) is less than 100 percent (witness the antismoking and seat belt compaigns), there have been some indications that individuals will change how they behave based on what we tell them.

The increasing concern with diet and exercise, the millions of joggers, marathon runners, swimmers, bikers, hikers, etc., crowding recreational facilities attest to the effectiveness of promotional efforts through books, sports broadcasts, lectures, and so on. Often the best that can be said of pure communication, however, is that it can bring people to the point of trying a behavior once, enhancing its psychological benefits, or reducing its social price. At some point, at least, the behaver must find the behavior worthwhile for it to be repeated.

It is difficult to estimate the true and total effects of communication. Behaviorists would tell us that behavior actually comes first, and attitudes follow. Most promotional efforts are aimed at identifying and changing attitudes so that behavior will follow. How much the din of advertising, the Chinese water torture of repeated messages, actually alters our thinking, knowledge, and behavior, as opposed to the results we experience from the behavior, is subject more to debate than conclusion.[2]

PROMOTING AWARENESS

The initial key to promotional efforts, like any marketing effort, is to have a specific behavior target in mind. If the target is to change the market's state of mind from unawareness to awareness, then you first must have a confident belief that the people you're aiming your efforts at are truly unaware of what you're trying to tell them about. The market audit or specific market research

[2] R. Cunningham, "Health Promotion: Forty Years of Trial, Error," *Hospitals, JAHA*, Dec. 1, 1978, p. 35.

results should tell you their current state of mind. You should not propose to pursue changes in the knowledge individuals have about your organization unless you know what their current knowledge is and what you'd like their future knowledge to be.

A promotional effort aimed at increasing knowledge should emphasize facts that are likely to concern and be used by markets in making the kinds of action decisions or choices you wish them to make. To design the proper focus for the message, you must understand what kinds of information people use in making such decisions, and provide it. In effect, this simply is an extension or corollary of the basic marketing approach of discovering what benefits people want to buy/use and delivering them.

There are not many instances in which individuals would alter their behavior simply on the basis of obtaining a new piece of knowledge, of course. The factors under which this might be true, however, include:

- people newly arrived in the area who have no knowledge or awareness of what services are available, and where, when, how, and from whom they may be obtained
- tourists or passersby who may have an emergency and wish to find the nearest source of needed service
- persons whose home or work situation restricts their care seeking or gives them a strong preference for a specific area of location or time of availability
- your development of a new service that you are offering for the first time to a current or new market (segment)

Each of these circumstances involves specific services and/or specific market segments to which you probably should tailor your message. New arrivals are likely to be looking for a permanent source of care as often as they are seeking an immediate expedient. What you tell them should emphasize the range of services you provide, the different family members to whom they are open, and the times they are available. Such messages probably should be repeated or displayed permanently as constant cues, since you can't know when they'll be making their first choice.

Information on your services, strictly facts without persuasion, can be communicated to this segment through brochures distributed by Welcome Wagon or Newcomers Groups. Mailings to new accounts at local utilities are another possibility. Stickers containing emergency phone numbers, including that of your organization, can be distributed as permanent reminders. Another possibility is calendars or maps—documents that newcomers might consult often and, if imprinted with short bits of information about your organization, keep their level of awareness high.

Tourists and other passersby make choices on availability and proximity, primarily. To communicate to them, you should emphasize passive, permanent displays. Some alternatives are covers for phone books in motel/hotel rooms, lobby displays, placards in taxicabs, etc. The highway department in most states provides signs pointing to the nearest hospital, and hospital emergency rooms use well-lit, large signs indicating their location. Care must be taken in some organizations where vivid displays announcing their location may dissuade people from entering (e.g., family planning, alcohol or drug care programs, abortion clinics, etc.)

Some emergency services, such as poison information or suicide prevention centers, can justify prominent displays in phone books, on buses or subways, as placards in public places, etc. Where these services are sponsored by larger organizations, they serve as a constant reminder to passersby, newcomers and the general public as to the name of the organization and the kinds of services it provides. Here, too, care must be taken not to overemphasize programs that might carry unsavory overtones to the general public.

Where individuals' home or work situations suggest a strong preference for an unusual time or specific location in which you offer services, and they are unaware that you do so, a repeated/permanent promotional effort is suggested. Messages can be conveyed through their employers via bulletin boards at work, and reminders can be included in pay envelopes or in their company publications. Where location is a choice factor, information on your organization's services can be posted at shopping centers, churches, or any other frequent gathering places for the community.

The key to segment-specific knowledge promotion is to identify the segment, tailor your message to the information its members will use, and make sure it reaches them as close as possible to the time they will use it to make a market decision. Perhaps a classic example of this principle is the story of an enterprising physician. As part of his market analysis, he recognized that the expanding volume of malpractice suits, considered a major crisis by most of his peers, also was a market opportunity. Such expansion meant an increasing number of persons who would need the services of a medical expert who could testify on their behalf that malpractice had occurred.

Such expanding demand for a product entailed little opposition. Most physicians continue to be reluctant to testify against their colleagues, preferring to handle problems of incompetence or misbehavior privately rather than in court. Thus, the expanding market for expert testimony was not attracting many other suppliers. By contacting and working out fees with other physicians around the country, the enterprising practitioner was able to offer his product nationally. Having identified a market, developed a product and place, and set a price, all that remained was to communicate to the interested public.

A general mailing served to communicate to the public at large the availability of this new service. However, the average person has a very low probability of being involved in a malpractice situation, and unless the mailing coincided fairly closely to the time of need, might not even remember the mailing. In an effort to focus communication on the proper segment at a propitious time, lists of all discharges from hospitals were obtained and brochures distributed to discharged patients, suggesting that if they had complaints about how they were treated, a malpractice service would be available to them.

Even this effort was not focused optimally. By obtaining lists of persons who already had instituted malpractice suits against hospitals, communication could be directed at precisely the market segment most receptive to the information at precisely the opportune time. The story goes that offers were made to hospital administrators to pass on the identity of persons suing the hospital so that their specific market segments could be identified accurately in a timely fashion. Whether this is true or whether anyone took advantage of an offer to split the testimony fee for "customers" referred is not clear, but the story illustrates two principles:

1. Communication of facts should be directed at precisely the market segments most interested in them at precisely the time when they can best use the information.
2. Promotional activities in the health care field are not governed by the same rules as elsewhere.

These events would be frowned upon in health care but applauded as enterprising and imaginative promotion in most other industries.

IMAGE BUILDING

While knowledge-focused communications efforts should be aimed at specific segments at precise times, general image-building communications usually are geared to the general public and repeated over extended periods. Usually, no specific behavior target or market segment is in mind for such communications, although some attitude and eventually behavior changes presumably are desired.

Even general image building should start from a known situation. To create a new or strengthen an existing opinion the public may have of your organization, you first must know what that opinion is. The market audit specifically should provide you with this information, which you can use to formulate your communications strategy and evaluate any results. Lacking a "before" picture, you'd have no way of knowing whether you had an image problem, how great it was, or what impact it might have on behavior that concerned you: voting, donations, utilization, etc.

There are a number of ways in which you can get messages to the general public in an effort to improve or modify your reputation. In marketing terminology, a sharp distinction is made between advertising and publicity:

- Advertising covers messages you design and pay for, delivered via signs, matchbook covers, newspaper, radio, or television.
- Publicity covers information others design and publish, delivered through media they control.

Advertising includes the sign on your building and individual notices within your facility—anything you write and pay for. It can include:

- placards posted in shopping centers
- annual reports sent out with Sunday newspapers
- brochures and other mailings
- radio or television spot announcements
- newspaper advertisements
- notices posted in taxis, buses, trains
- signs on the highway

The chief advantages of advertising lie in the control you have over exactly what message is communicated through what medium. The disadvantages lie in the fact that you have to pay for it, that you may run into ethical issues, and that your message may not have high credibility when people recognize your authorship.

Publicity includes everything others say or write about you, through whatever media they use. It can include:

- news stories about famous people being treated by you, or just visiting patients
- news stories about accident or disaster victims cared for by your organization
- announcements of meetings, fairs, screening programs, events taking place in your organization
- negative stories regarding malpractice suits, scandals, or other newsworthy internal problems

The chief advantage of publicity is that it is free and is published through more objective, higher credibility sources. The major disadvantage is your lack of control over what is communicated.

In practice, the distinction between advertising and publicity often is blurred as your organization attempts to exploit its advantages and minimize its disadvantages. You can pay to have developed public information messages on health hazards or health behavior and have them delivered free as public service announcements by television and radio. A good example of this strategy is described in Chapter 16. You may pay to put on a health fair or free screening program or other public service whose existence will be publicized at no cost to you by the media. You may pay the expenses for a well-known figure to visit your organization, address a meeting, etc., as a means of getting your organization's name in the newspaper.

It is a common practice in public relations to measure the effectiveness of these efforts in terms of column inches of newspaper space, minutes of air time, or other media messages devoted to the organization. Marketing would insist that this is merely an intermediate measure, an interim device suggesting what your behavior is, and reserve judgment to see what impacts can be tied to it. Unless you have some idea what kinds of behavior you eventually hope your communications promote, you may be spending a lot of money, time, and effort on nothing, or not enough to achieve anything significant. It is difficult to tie "image building" to specific behavior in practice, but you ought at least to have a link between them in mind.

ACTION

It is a truism that "action speaks louder than words." This applies equally to the promotion of health care organizations or programs. Whether your target is a specific behavior change in a specific market segment, or the general public attitude toward your organization, you don't have to rely on words to get your message across. In many ways, your actions will serve to reinforce or even substitute for verbal messages and are likely to have stronger effects than mere words. If one picture is worth a thousand words, then one action is equal to at least a few pictures.

When you are asking persons who are relatively unaware of your existence or your programs to become aware, interested, and finally to decide to use your services, you can encourage this transition by your own action. A screening program, for example, especially one taken to where people are and delivered at little or no cost to them, can accomplish two major purposes: (1) It can make people aware they have conditions requiring health services that you provide (hypertension, vision/hearing, diabetes, V.D., cancer). (2)

It also will remind individuals that you are concerned with their health, that you exist, and that you offer services.

To attract new markets, or old markets to new services, you may offer tours through your facility or maintain booths in shopping malls describing your services staffed by volunteers willing to talk about them. By arranging personal contact with prospective markets, you can enhance the effectiveness of your verbal messages significantly. Where you have a specific market segment in mind, you should tailor your action so as to maximize that group's awareness of it, so you can benefit from it wherever possible.

To get possible customers to become acquainted with your facility, you may host health-related or even unrelated community services. These include prenatal classes hosted by hospitals, continuing education for physicians or referral agency personnel, and meetings of local professional and civic organizations. By hosting such events, first you get individuals to visit your organization and, potentially, be impressed by your existence and any other positive observable attributes, and second, you express your public spirit and concern with community health.

The hosting of such events serves the additional function of increasing the likelihood and frequency of your being mentioned by the media. Announcements of these events in many cases will be made through radio and/or television, and reports carried in newspapers. While hosting meetings or other group events may entail some expense to you, it is likely to be an effective source of good-will and image-building publicity. Where the event is related specifically to a service you provide, so much the better, since it will establish or reinforce a connection in the public mind. The general challenge of establishing and maintaining the desired image, or psychological market position, is discussed in Chapter 9.

SERVICE BEHAVIOR

The most effective means of communication regarding the availability and acceptability of health services seems always to have been word-of-mouth advertising. To make maximum use of this medium, you should concentrate a fair amount of attention on your own service behavior. In effect, you should increase to a maximum the probability that individuals will be saying good things about you. Unlike other "advertising," you can't absolutely control what people will say, but you should devote some effort to understanding, predicting, and influencing such behavior.

One suggestion that arises from previous discussion is that you should try to learn what people are saying about you—not merely their attitudes or knowledge, but what they are communicating and to whom about your organization. Your market audit, or service-specific market research is, again, a potential source of this information. You will have to ask people what they hear and from whom (your employees, medical staff, board members, volunteers, patients) as well as what they tell others. This is a particularly good reason for using an outside, objective agency to conduct such research, to increase the probability of getting accurate responses.

If you find the messages being communicated via word of mouth are less than what you'd like, you are likely to have to change your behavior in order to change individuals' stories. Complaints about your product, place, or price cannot be eliminated by your verbal messages. If your food is cold and unpalatable, you will have to address the problem rather than "jam" communications with your own ideas of how good your food is.

One particularly adroit approach to this problem is being used by at least one hospital (see Chapter 16). One of its regular publications is devoted specifically and entirely to comments by patients on the care they received. Where the comments are positive, the specific employee(s) cited for praise are reported for all to read. Where comments are negative (rarely), only the department is reported, though the manager of that department is informed about the specific employee(s) named.

Such a program serves at least two purposes. It reminds employees of the importance the organization places on how patients are treated and feel about their care, rewarding through recognition those individuals who do a particularly good job of pleasing customers. It also should enhance the extent to which employees strive to please patients and improve the messages that both groups communicate to the public.

In general, employees are likely to be most critical of the quality of care your organization provides. This may be because of a perfectionist professional attitude or partly to their greater awareness of the mistakes made. Your employees also are likely to be considered the most reliable source of information about your services. This dangerous combination should be addressed consciously in your personnel policies as well as in your promotional planning. The second most credible source of data to the public about your organization is your patients. In addition to your attempts to understand, predict, and influence their use of services, you should ensure they are disseminating the kinds of messages you want.

Physicians and referral agencies are a special case of word-of-mouth advertising. What they think and say about you are likely to be very important factors in affecting their behavior as well as that of their colleagues. They are not always a particularly strong source of messages to the public because of their sensitivity about talking shop to outsiders. Their communication to their patients, your employees, and their colleagues, however, may tend toward the critical also for the same reasons as your employees. You must be especially sensitive to the kinds of messages they are communicating and govern your behavior accordingly.

SUMMARY

Promotion is a sufficiently important, though subservient, factor in marketing to merit special attention. It is by definition the communication of information to your publics and markets that you hope will influence their attitudes and behavior. It has limited scope, however, based on the extent to which information, by itself, is capable of altering individuals' knowledge, attitude, or behavior. It fits in marketing after the first three Ps, since it concerns itself mainly with informing people about your product, place, and price, although it also may be used under the label "health education" to promote changes in the public's health behavior generally.

Promoting awareness or knowledge of your organization is one function of communications efforts. To obtain the maximum effects, those efforts should be focused on a specific market segment and timed as closely as possible to when individuals will use the information you provide in making a market decision. Separate messages, media, and timing are likely to be necessary for distinct market segments. Care must be taken to be sure the messages are factual and the media acceptable for the unique characteristics of the health industry.

Image building is another major purpose of promotional efforts. They involve more general messages, repeated rather than timed, and aimed at the public at large rather than specific market segments. Either advertising (you pay for what you say) or publicity (you don't pay for what they say)—or both—may be used in promotional efforts. The two may be combined through public service messages, announcements, or sponsored events. The ultimate test of effectiveness of your promotional efforts should be significant, measured changes in your image—what people know or feel about you—and ultimately, the promise of changes in behavior.

Action is a separate but related promotional strategy. It can include sponsoring screening or simple services to reach out to your community, conducting tours or arranging exhibits, hosting meetings or educational programs, or newsworthy events. Both the personal contact with your organization this promotes and the publicity that results from such actions serve useful promotional purposes.

The way you serve your markets is ultimately the most effective promotional strategy. By being sensitive to and responding to concerns of your patients, employees, physicians, volunteers, and board members, you can increase the likelihood that the messages being spread via word-of-mouth advertising are helpful to you. You should identify current messages and monitor changes over time to ensure that your efforts in this direction are successful. Separate approaches are likely to be useful for each distinct segment of persons who may either recommend or discourage other markets.

Readings

Health Journals

Blaine, R. "What Makes a Successful Hospital Marketing Program." *Hospital Public Relations* 3:7, July 1977, p. 1.

"Bromberg Says Poll Emphasizes Need to Tell Public Why Hospital Costs Have Increased." *FAH Review,* July 1977, p. 10.

De Noyer, J. "Hospitals Seek Ways of Relating to Communities." *Hospitals, JAHA,* April 1, 1977, p. 127.

"Hospitals Learn Marketing Techniques." *Hospital Public Relations* 4:6, June 1978, p. 1.

"How Tennessee Hospitals Are Winning Community Support." *Opinion Leader News,* Spring 1977, p. 1.

Karr, D. "Increasing a Hospital's Market Share." *Hospitals, JAHA* 51, June 1, 1977, p. 64.

Marshall, C. "Ethical Aspects of Advertising Debated," *Modern Healthcare,* 7:4, April 1977, p. 48.

Ralston, R. "Hospital Advertiser Denies Existence of Marketing Program." *Modern Healthcare,* October 1977, p. 70.

Rescola, W. "Give Your Public the Straight Story on Hospital Costs." *Trustee,* June 1977, p. 36.

Sparber, P. "Hospital Public Relations—Is It Manageable?" *Hospital Financial Management,* January 1978, p. 18.

Ziff, D. "Community Relations: Hospitals Engage in Educational, Marketing Efforts." *Hospitals, JAHA,* 52:7, April 1, 1978, p. 69.

Nonhealth Journals

Cialdini, R. "A Test of Two Techniques for Inducing Verbal Behavioral, and Further Compliance with a Request to Give Blood." Working paper, Tempe, Ariz.: Arizona State University.

Cialdini, R., et al. "Reciprocal Concessions Procedure for Inducing Compliance." *Journal of Personality and Social Psychology* 31, February 1975, p. 206.

Hovland, C., and Weiss, W. "The Influence of Source Credibility on Communicator Effectiveness." *Public Opinion Quarterly* 15, Winter 1951-52, p. 635.

Miller, R., et al. "Attribution vs. Persuasion as a Means for Modifying Behavior." *Journal of Personality and Social Psychology* 31, March 1975, p. 430.

Scott, C. "The Effects of Trial and Incentives on Repeat Purchase Behavior." *Journal of Marketing Research* 13, August 1976, p. 263.

Sternthal, B., et al. "The Persuasive Effect of Source Credibility." *Public Opinion Quarterly,* Summer 1978, p. 64.

Tybout, A. "Relative Effectiveness of Three Behavioral Influence Strategies as Supplements to Persuasion in a Marketing Context." *Journal of Marketing Research* XV, May 1978, p. 229.

Health Education

Avery, C., et al. "Reducing Emergency Visits of Asthmatics: An Experiment in Patient Education." Paper presented at a hearing of the President's Committee on Health, Pittsburgh, 1972.

The Community Health Education Project—Final Report, Washington, D.C.: American Public Health Association, 1976.

Disease Control and Health Education and Promotion, Hearing before the Subcommittee on Health of the Committee on Labor and Public Welfare, U.S. Senate, May 7-8, 1975, Washington, D.C.: U.S. Government Printing Office, 1975.

Inui, T. "Doctor Education Leads to Effective Patient Education." *Health Education Report* 1:3, March-April 1974, p. 7.

A Survey of Consumer Health Education Programs, Cambridge, Mass.: Arthur D. Little, Inc., 1976.

"Making Health Education Work," *American Journal of Public Health* 65:10, Supplement, October 1975.

Morhouse, L., and Gross, L. *Total Fitness in Thirty Minutes a Week.* New York: Simon & Schuster, 1975.

Robbins, Lewis, and Hall, Jack. *How to Practice Prospective Medicine,* Indianapolis: Methodist Hospital of Indiana Health Hazards Appraisal Program, 1970.

Rosenstock, I., and Kirscht, J. "Practice Implications in the Health Belief Model and Personal Health Behavior." *Health Education Monographs* 2:4, Winter 1974, p. 470.

Chapter 8

Priority Setting

The job of rating or ranking competing choices in priority order is an ever-present challenge in any decision-making or management activity. It is equally as important in marketing. Despite its common use and importance, however, there is anything but a universal notion as to what priority means, and no generally accepted method for setting priorities. Both issues of meaning and questions of technique, and more particularly their interaction, are evaluated in this chapter.

MEANING

Before analyzing methods for determining the priority of competing choices, or the application of such ranking in marketing, it should be useful to consider priority's meaning. What do we mean when we rate items as "high priority?" If we rank a series of choices from one to ten, is it clear to everyone concerned how their behavior should differ toward No. 7 vs. No. 6? Do we do the high-priority items first or just try to do them better? There are five distinguishable ways we might intend priority to be interpreted into action. However, these are not necessarily consistent with each other:

1. rhetorical priority
2. sequential priority
3. quantitative priority
4. qualitative priority
5. all-or-nothing priority

Rhetorical Priority

The most common meaning of priority is purely rhetorical, or having no specified meaning in terms of action. We talk about high-priority problems or goals as a way of indicating the extent of our concern over them. Until and unless we have analyzed choices more thoroughly, however, we simply haven't made up our minds how we intend to behave. By assigning a label of high priority to an item, we pretend we've given it the attention it deserves, knowing we haven't yet given it enough attention to know precisely how individuals should behave toward it. It is like saluting a statue—a gesture of respect but one we won't let interfere with our normal behavior.

Rhetorical priority can serve a useful purpose, however. Considering the large number of interests that may be competing for your organization's attention, rhetorical statements of priority may communicate at least the depth of your concern. Unless your expression is followed up with some action eventually, however, your communications may not keep such interests happy very long. For external groups that aren't aware of or don't care exactly how you operate your priorities, you may be able to satisfy expectations by giving out many No. 1 priority ratings and promising some meaningful action. Demonstrating the exact effect of priority rating on your behavior may be unnecessary and even meaningless to external publics.

Sequential Priority

Sequential priority expresses an intention to get to higher priority items earlier, and the highest priority issue first. Given this definition or operational translation of priority, you obviously should consider where being first makes a significant difference. For items of extremely high importance, it may even be necessary to determine that they will be completed first, not merely begun early. A specific target date may then be a more meaningful expression of your intention than the priority label per se.

Unfortunately, it is by no means always true that what has to or should be done first is high priority in any other way. Some things have to be done first simply because they are required for some logical sequence. Some things *are* carried out first merely because some additional planning or preparation must be done before you can get on with what's really important. You may do first the things that are easiest, or require an obvious and small amount of resources, just to get them out of the way. Such a temporal priority may signify nothing in the way of rhetorical or any other kind of priority.

Quantitative Priority

A quantitative interpretation of priority suggests that higher priority items receive more resources: more time and attention, more effort, more funds. This is somewhat like paying the most for what's most important to you. It would tend to be accepted readily as a validation or demonstration that you mean your priorities, putting your money where your mouth is. At face value, it would appear clear that if something is most important or highest priority, it deserves the most.

Unfortunately, this logic is flawed. What is most important may not be amenable to use of the largest share of your resources. Unless the situation of most importance is one that also can benefit from a strategy whose implementation requires the greatest share, automatic translation of priority into quantity of resources allocated could waste resources. There is no particular reason to assume that this will occur any more than coincidentally. Whatever the rhetorical value of putting your resources where your priorities are, the practical consequences may not be what you'd like at all.

Qualitative Priority

Another perfectly logical translation of priority would be to assign your best resources to your highest priorities—your best equipment, most effective personnel, and so on. This would be accepted in most cases as a reasonable reflection of the importance you attach to a situation: "I'll put my best person on it." Because you are promising only quality, not quantity, you can gear the amount of your best resources to the amount the situation can use rather than be trapped into giving it the most. If it is truly the most important area, the employment of your best resources should promise the best possible outcome.

Such an approach has to be used carefully, however. What may be your highest quality resources may not be most appropriate to the situation. Your most senior personnel may not have as much specific competence and experience relative to a given problem as one of your more junior. However, if you select as best those resources most appropriate to the situation, the combination of best and highest priority may be a reasonable and effective way to translate priority operationally. Such a coupling may serve to reward your best personnel, for example, since those experts are given the most important assignments.

All-or-Nothing Priority

This unusual approach to priorities says, in effect, that No. 1 priority is so important compared to others that all available resources will be used up for it before you go on to No. 2. If No. 1 priority can benefit reasonably from all the resources at your disposal, then none are left over for No. 2. If the first one can't really use all you have, you can allocate what remains to No. 2, and so forth. This translation means that whatever is necessary and can be applied to a higher priority will be applied before a lower priority gets any allocation.

Such an operational definition of priority rarely is appropriate—the Manhattan Project in World War II comes to mind as an example of its use—but may occur for extremely high priority issues. The greatest risk lies in assuming that only large and inflexible amounts of resources can be of any use. The Hill-Burton priorities for hospital construction gave whatever was needed to high priority before giving any to lower. The possibility of giving a little less than the total needed in order to be able to assist more projects could have been examined as an alternative. The risk of the all-or-nothing approach is that the costs of doing nothing about lower priority items may never be appreciated.

These five alternative translations of priority into action meanings no doubt do not exhaust the possibilities. However, they should point out the advisability of making sure you have in mind the meaning of priority you intend before you make priority assignments. There may be worlds of difference among the implications of rhetorical, sequential, quantitative, qualitative, and all-or-nothing translations in specific instances. It also would be advisable that the intended meaning of priority be made clear to those whose behavior is meant to be affected.

APPLICATIONS

Audit

The determination of priorities occurs in a substantial number of places throughout a marketing program. In designing and later implementing a market audit, potential items for inclusion have to be ranked in order to ensure that the most important are included. The only reason for setting priorities is the underlying assumption that you can't do everything, and therefore have to make some choices. In a market audit, the choice is whether or not to add more items of information given the cost vs. the benefit of doing so. Your priorities should be assigned from the perspective of knowing there is a limit to how much information you can collect; how much time, effort, and money you can spend on the project; and how long you can wait for results. If you are using an incremental strategy for developing the audit, this means keeping the first version fairly simple.

You may design your priorities around specific information targets: inside vs. outside, patients vs. physicians, outpatients vs. inpatients, for example. Thus you would attempt to learn more about your high-priority market segments. Another way of segmenting the audit for priority setting would be to use its structure: impacts vs. behavior, behavior vs. causes. A third approach would be to ensure that you learn a little about everything and plan a more in-depth effort later. In this way, you are using more of a sequential meaning of priority than implying what's most important.

The sequential is probably the easiest translation of priority. While it indicates what you plan to do first, it doesn't say when you plan to get to second. If the information you discover in your first audit truly is threatening or promising, you may begin your second, in-depth audit immediately. It may be a lot easier to decide, as a group, what should be done first rather than what's important. By translating priority into precise operational significance, you should increase the likelihood that agreement can be reached on priority rankings.

Another example of priority in the market audit is the level your markets place on specific product or price attributes. You may ask them to rank their major concerns or the services they feel they need most. One way of identifying the extent of preference is to ask potential customers how far they'd be willing to travel to obtain a specific service, how much they'd pay for it, or how long they'd be willing to wait for it. Their responses may well indicate their use of priority, though the frequency as well as intensity of their perceived need undoubtedly will enter into their thinking.

Physicians may be asked to rank their major complaints or needs. While you don't have to follow their preferences slavishly, you'd be better off at least knowing what they are. Similar analysis is possible on employee preferences (e.g., Herzberg's satisfiers vs. dissatisfiers), board members, volunteers, etc. How you respond to these preferences is your choice, but being able to see things from their perspective should help you.

Problems, Threats, Opportunities

The results of the market audit also will suggest some priority ranking. Each problem or threat or opportunity should be ranked against others of its type on the basis of sequence, quantitative, or qualitative resource implications. You may wish to set priorities among the three, in general (all problems get addressed first, then threats, with opportunities last) or specific-to-the-individual cases of each. If the limited amount of resources available and the need to do something first are recognized, priority may reflect any one or more of the five alternative meanings discussed previously.

You may assign priorities differently for different phases of your marketing program. In analyzing problems, threats, and opportunities, you may assign the highest priority for analysis to the most severe or significant in terms of impact, expecting that the analysis will reveal two other important factors: the probability of impact and the feasibility of intervention. On the basis of your analysis, you may decide then which problems, threats, or opportunities should be given high priority for action. Since this latter priority reflects additional factors, it probably will not be the same as your initial priorities for analysis.

GOALS AND OBJECTIVES

Like problems, threats, and opportunities, priority rankings among market goals and objectives should be based on multiple factors. These include, at a minimum, the desirability of change (how good the impact would be), the probability of change (how likely it is to occur) and the feasibility of your intervention (whether legally or financially possible). A goal may be stated entirely on the basis of its desirability. Objectives should be adopted formally only after analysis of probability and feasibility.

Priorities among goals often may be rhetorical, since they are based on desirability alone. Objectives always must be practical, so priorities should reflect sequential or resource allocation meanings. Initial priorities among goals may indicate simply which ones you're going to analyze first, which you'll see about setting objectives and developing strategies for this year vs. next. Your analysis then should indicate which goals are most amenable to pursuit or most capable of achievement. Once you know that, you can decide which merit specific objectives and strategies in what priority order.

Objectives should be ranked only after you have analyzed the value of their impact as well as the probability of successful implementation of the strategies that will achieve the objective. If you can evaluate competing objectives in terms of the same measurable impact (financial viability, health status index), you can rank them on a purely quantitative basis. The cost vs. the impact of each should provide a simple mathematical ranking. The meaning of the ranking is still more important than the process used to develop it, especially if you can't measure competing objectives in similar terms.

STRATEGIES

Once objectives have been identified on a draft basis, or often before objectives are even considered, you may be examining alternative actions. Alternatives always exist, even if they are go vs. no-go decisions. Priority ranking among alternative action decisions may indicate which you will implement and which you won't. In many cases, priority may indicate which actions you will try first, retaining the others as fallback possibilities if the approvals or resources necessary to implement your first choice aren't forthcoming.

The basis for selecting among competing action alternatives always should be the cost vs. the benefit of each compared to the others. You may be assigning your priorities from one of two different situations:

1. fixed objectives or
2. fixed resources

For a fixed objective, you know what absolutely must be accomplished—the essential outcome—so strategies can be rated according to how well each promises to achieve the necessary result. Each strategy should have the same basic benefit: achieving your essential outcome. Therefore, each can be priority ordered or preference ranked according to the cost. In reality, it's a little more complicated. Each may produce some side effects, some of which may be benefits and others costs (the product vs. the price of each to you). You then will have to pick the best bargain.

For fixed resources, you know how much you have available to spend (time, money, personnel, etc.) and can rank alternative actions based on how much benefit each would promise for the same cost. Again, alternatives are likely to have side effects that have to be thrown into the balance. The probability as well as the value of each impact has to be considered. The same goes for costs.

Formal decision analysis (decision trees) may be used in this analysis. In simplest form, this means evaluating strategies mathematically based on the probability times the impact value of each. If you can estimate that strategy A will produce net revenues of $50,000 and has a probability of .50 of being successful, then it would be preferred to strategy B, which promises greater net revenues ($100,000) but has much lower probability of success (.10). The preference of each is expressed as:

A $50,000 × .50 = $25,000

B $100,000 × .10 = $10,000

This obviously is an artificial construct, since in neither case will you actually get $25,000 or $10,000 net revenue. You'll get either $50,000, $100,000, or nothing. It may well be difficult for you to evaluate the probability of each. By expending your best effort, however, you can provide some useful mathematical assistance to your decision process.

OUTCOMES

It is one thing to assign preferences to actions based on their expected outcomes—probability times impact value—but what do you do with actions you've taken already? Where outcomes are known, the response to them may not be as straightforward a decision as it seems. If a program you've implemented produces only half the value you expected, do you cut its budget as a punishment or increase its budget to promote full achievement? Where another program has overfilled its quota or produced more value than you expected, do you increase its budget as a reward, or cut it back in recognition that it needs less?

Such decisions have important morale as well as financial consequences. Rewarding an unsuccessful program by increasing its budget and punishing a successful one by decreases may not be well accepted by the personnel directly involved or elsewhere in the organization. Yet budget allocations, especially changes from year to year, are likely to be interpreted as direct reflections of your priorities. If you don't intend them that way, you should make clear to your publics exactly what budget changes signify.

The "solution" to this dilemma is to ignore the past, the accomplishment vs. expectation reward or punishment (except for morale implications). Any resource allocation to an existing program is a marginal change and should be evaluated in terms of marginal impact. How much more benefit will you get by allocating more resources to one program (quantitative priority) than another? How much more benefit will you derive out of increasing a program's budget vs. keeping it the same or reducing it? Is the cost vs. the benefit for one change better than another?

In effect, you are a consumer with fixed resources making buying decisions in a market. You have to decide what purchases will provide you with the greatest utilities (product) for their overall cost (price). Each is a new purchase and to be decided upon based on expected future benefits. Your expectations should arise from past performance, but you're not trying to reward past behavior as much as derive the most possible value out of the future. Your buyer's preference (priority) should reflect your changing needs and values as well as the promised outcomes of your alternative choices.

METHODS

A number of methodological issues in priority setting for different applications have been described in passing. The method used to set priorities should take into account the meaning of priority in operational terms and the persons whose behavior is to be affected by the rankings. Whatever method is chosen, it should include identification of specific factors to be considered, weighting of such factors, and some way of summing the combination to evaluate competing choices.

The simplest form of priority ranking is the *group consensus* approach. Basically, it involves asking a group of concerned persons to rank choices as they see them. The implications of the ranking should be clear, but no precise factors or weights are employed. In effect, all participants use their own evaluation approach and simply arrive at a consensus. This may be achieved informally through discussion or formally via some voting process. Each may rank each alternative, with the final rankings derived from the average of the group. Such an approach is fine when you either don't care what factors the group uses in making its judgment (e.g., rhetorical priority) or you are confident in its use of appropriate factors, or perhaps when you have no choice.

A formal *weighting matrix* may be useful in some circumstances. Specific factors are identified, recognizing that they must be considered in making a priority or action preference decision. Here again, the meaning and operational implications must be made clear before such factors are identified. Each factor then is weighted, based on its importance. Each choice then is evaluated against the others on each factor. The value assigned each choice is multiplied by the weight for each factor, then the scores of each choice are derived via adding or even multiplying individual scores. A simple example of this approach is illustrated in Figure 8-1.

Figure 8-1 A Weighting Matrix for Setting Priorities

Factors	Strategies			
	A	**B**	**C**	
Cost (highest = 0, lowest = 10)	$7/49$	$5/35$	$2/10$	Unweighted score
Weight = 7				Weighted score
Benefit (highest = 10, lowest = 0)	$4/20$	$6/30$	$8/40$	
Weight = 5				
Feasibility (highest = 10, lowest = 0)	$9/27$	$3/9$	$1/3$	
Weight = 3				
Summed score (weighted)	96	74	53	
Multiplied score (weighted)	26,460	9,450	1,200	

Note: Multiplied scores often are different from summed scores, so the choice is a significant one.

According to the figure, strategy A clearly is the first choice, whether summed or multiplied scores are used. Your own judgment will have to tell you whether the factors best fit summed or multiplied. When a factor representing feasibility or probability is used, a multiplication often makes more sense. This will enable you to wipe out an alternative that has a feasibility or probability of zero. Otherwise, you might find yourself preferring a choice that is admirable in all respects but impossible to implement or is purely theoretical.

The particular example in Figure 8-1 is a *fixed-range* scale and weighting system with both high and low scores fixed. Other permutations include fixing the high only or low only, or fixing neither. Ranks rather than weights and scores may be used, but tend not to distinguish clearly between widely different strategies since the best never is more than one number away from the second best. A group consensus approach may be used in conjunction with the formal matrix, such as by having the group average weights and scores and ratify results. For simplicity, unweighted factors may be used if they are considered sufficiently similar in importance.

Each of these methods is designed to be an aid to judgment, not a substitute for it. If the group is the decision-making body, it may employ consensus instead of or in addition to a formal analytical process. If the group is merely advisory, additional analyses may be performed. In any case, the reasons for setting priority (e.g., limited resources), the implications of ranking on behavior, and the full effects of both the choices and the ranking must be identified and considered for effective priority setting.

SUMMARY

Priorities often must be set among choices competing for your attention or resources. In going about the task of priority setting, it is essential that the meaning of priority—its implications for behavior—be identified. Priority may have purely rhetorical meaning, expressing your values but not guiding your behavior. It may translate into where you assign your best resources, the most, or simply what you work on first. In extreme circumstances, it may identify where all your effort will be directed. The logic of translation into behavior as well as the basis for establishing priorities deserve careful and explicit attention.

Priority setting may be applied in any or all of a large number of situations in a marketing program. Ranking of information items in your market audit will indicate which are to be included in early editions. Priority among problems, threats, and opportunities first should guide your analysis and subsequently your action, though different factors will be considered and different priorities result for the two. Priorities among goals should express your values, while ranking of objectives reflects your confident expectations as well. Choosing among strategies is a special application of priorities, since it tends to focus on selecting one rather than ranking all alternatives. Rating outcomes is another special case, important for its implications on, as well as interpretation by, specific programs.

There are basically two classes of priority-setting methods: group process and quantitative/analytical. The former may employ either formal or informal approaches, consensus, voting, or averaging ranks. The latter typically employs specific quantifiable factors of importance, with weights and scores for each. Final priority ranking then is calculated from the sum or product of factor scores. Group process and quantitative techniques may be combined, rather than relying exclusively on one. In any case, the final decision is a matter of your judgment.

Readings

Blum, H. "Priority Setting for Problems, Solutions and Projects by Means of Selected Criteria." *International Journal of Health Services* 2:1, February 1972, p. 85.

Blum, H. *Planning for Health.* New York: Human Sciences Press, 1974, Chapters 6 and 7, pp. 218-299.

Gentry, J. "The Planning of Community Health Services: Facilitating Rational Decision-Making." *Inquiry* 8, September 1971, p. 4.

Holder, L., and Deniston, L. "A Decision-Making Approach to Comprehensive Health Planning." *Public Health Reports* 83:7, July 1968, p. 559.

Kane, R. "Determination of Health Care Priorities and Expectations Among Rural Consumers." *Health Services Research* 4:2, Summer 1969, p. 142.

Locke, J. "Identifying Product-Safety Priorities." *Operations Research* 22:6, November-December 1974, p. 1206.

MacStravic, R. "Setting Priorities in Health Planning: What Does It All Mean?" *Inquiry* 15, March 1978, p. 20.

Richardson, J., and Scutchfield, F. "Priorities in Health Care." *American Journal of Public Health* 63:1, January 1973, p. 79.

Scutchfield, F. "Alternate Methods for Health Priority Assessment." *Journal of Community Health* 1:1, Fall 1975, p. 29.

Stimson, D. "Utility Measurement in Public Health Decision Making." In Reisman, A. and Kiley, M. *Health Care Delivery Planning,* New York, Gordon and Breach, 1973, p. 63.

Welsh, K. "Initiating Community Health Development in an Appalachian Community." *American Journal of Public Health* 58:7, July 1958, p. 1162.

Williamson, J. "Evaluating Quality of Patient Care: A Strategy Relating Outcome and Process Improvement." *JAMA* 218, October 25, 1971, p. 564.

Part III

Taking Action

Marketing audits and strategic analysis are designed to lead up to action—decisions and implementation. To make the best use of analytical techniques and results, they must be understood and employed in the context of the action toward which they point you. While marketing insists that you stand there and think a while before doing anything, it does not permit you merely to think about situations. Marketing focuses on changes in behavior—achieving them or preventing them. It assumes you have to make changes in yourself in order to alter your market relationships. It is an action-oriented discipline that employs systematic research and analysis as an introduction to (not a substitute for) the real story—taking action.

Four major categories of action decisions are discussed in Part III. Chapter 9 covers the most basic market decision of all: the choice and pursuit of a specific market position. The position you pursue will have both physical and psychological sides to it, from your own perspective as well as from that of your markets. Market positioning is designed to focus and build on your organization's strengths, the market's perceived needs, and your competition's weaknesses. If carried out effectively, it would ensure your organization's viability and significant contribution, and make government control of health services development superfluous.

The second type of market action, presented in Chapter 10, is that of the resource decision. Having decided on any effort in principle, how do you estimate the resources required to carry out that effort in practice? Resource decisions are necessary in analysis as part of estimating the cost vs. the benefit of particular actions. They are equally critical in implementation, since identifying and acquiring necessary resources are essential steps in overall management. The model for resource decisions in this chapter specifically incorporates marketing techniques and market analysis inputs in its basic approach. While only two examples are provided, the model can be and has been used for all kinds of health resource decisions.

The third type of action, covered in Chapter 11, involves the design and execution of a marketing management approach. It describes the necessary and optimal relationships between marketing and five critical components of the health organization. It offers suggestions that you can use to build such linkages and explains why they are necessary. It helps answer questions on what specifically you should do and how you should behave in order to have an effective marketing program. It should help you fit marketing, both conceptually and practically, into the kind of health organization in which you're working.

Finally, in Chapter 12, problems, issues, and techniques of marketing marketing are discussed. To introduce an effective marketing program, you have to be able to design and promote the kind of program you have in mind. Your program must meet the expectations of its markets within your organization if it is to be supported and accepted by those it affects. Specific ethical issues, potential sources of resistance, arguments, and techniques you can use are presented.

Chapter 9

Marketing Positioning

Possibly the single most important concept in marketing is that of market positioning. By definition, your market position is simply the mix of products you provide to the mix of people who use them. It is what you do with whom, the set of market relationships you actually have, with patients, physicians, and whoever else you choose to view from a marketing perspective. It has two separate though related forms: your actual market position and your reputed market position. The first is measured in terms of facts: what types and amounts of products you actually provide to what types and numbers of individuals. The second is measured in terms of psychographics: what people think you are and do.

In the past, determination of market position by health care organizations has been carried out primarily through two nonmarketing philosophies:

1. the determination of what the community needs and the acceptance of a moral obligation to respond to those needs
2. the insistence on being and doing the best in whatever the organization does as a matter of pride as well as obligation

NEED AND PRIDE

Perhaps the most dangerous practice in health care development has been its characteristic insistence on responding to need. In health care, it is the professionals who define need, each with a slightly different perspective. Once it is believed that residents in the community need a service, the organization accepts its obligation to respond to that need and develops the facilities, equipment, and personnel resources required to do so. On the surface, this is a laudable philosophy and has made it difficult to employ effective marketing.

111

Some apologists for marketing insist that it, too, is a discipline attempting to identify and respond to human needs. If it were, the health field could claim to have been doing exemplary marketing throughout its existence. In fact, however, marketing is a discipline that attempts to predict, influence, and respond to how individuals behave. The difference is significant, even though it may strip the marketing field of some of its righteous patina.

Professionally defined need, in effect, identifies how people ought to behave and how the organization ought to accommodate that behavior. It is normal practice to view health care transactions from the provider's perspective: *delivering* health services, *rendering* care, *providing* counseling, *delivering* babies. Each transaction has its flip side, however: *utilizing* health services, *receiving* care, *accepting* counseling, *presenting* babies for obstetricians to "catch." There is no correct way to view these transactions. Both groupings are perfectly valid and equally descriptive. There can be no delivery without receiving, no doctoring without patienting, no counseling without clients, no nursing without patients, etc.

Marketing specifically recognizes the two-part nature of such transactions and insists that both be analyzed as part of development. The nonmarketing approach common to health care says in effect:

- They need it.
- We'll provide it.
- They should come.
- We should prosper.

Marketing employs an asking rather than a telling approach:

- What will they use?
- What can we best provide?
- How many will come?
- Would we prosper?

The essence of market positioning is to answer these questions as objectively and accurately as possible and make development decisions accordingly. Health care organizations for years have been exempt from the necessity of effective market positioning because of their unique market.

- Health insurance increasingly has insulated the consumer from the direct financial impact of health services use while ensuring providers that they will be paid whatever is used.
- Health care financing in public organizations and hospitals has been geared to reimbursing costs, thus protecting programs that are overbuilt or underused from direct fiscal consequences.

- Hospitals have accepted the necessity of continuing some programs that operate at a loss (obstetrics, pediatrics) because of need, while covering such losses with the gains from other programs (laboratory, x-ray, pharmacy).

All these factors are targeted for change, especially the last two. Under many of the national health insurance proposals, consumers will have to pay part of the costs of each service through either deductibles or coinsurance requirements. Cost-based reimbursement for publicly funded programs is threatened by taxpayer revolt, while it is on the way out in most states for hospitals. Nursing homes have long been told what their costs should be, and hospitals have begun to join them, thanks to rate-setting and rate-review commissions. Cross-subsidization of services also is being attacked and its demise is specifically called for in Section 1533 of the National Health Planning and Resources Development Act of 1974 (P.L. 93-641).

What these changes will mean to health care organizations is that they will have to begin to operate under the same rules as most other industries have throughout their existence. Health care organizations will have to identify and achieve a viable market position in order to survive. No longer will they be able to do what they think is best for their community; they'll have to focus on what they can afford to do and on what people will and can afford to use. No longer will they be able to insist on the best of everything; they'll have to consider seriously what the community can afford, both in quantity and quality of care.

In effect, consumers are being replaced by planning and regulatory agencies as judges of what their needs are and what they can afford. For some years, the health care system has been able to act on what it decided people need while the larger community has gotten stuck with the bill. Now the larger community is saying that if we pay, we say. Certificate of need, Utilization Review, Appropriateness Review, and Professional Services Review Organizations all are efforts to substitute wider, public-oriented judgments of what should be done by whom for individual provider decisions.

It is unlikely that direct efforts will be made to regulate what the individual consumer demands and the individual provider decides is appropriate in the use of services. Rather, capital expenditure controls and operational expenditure limits will put a lid on how much will be paid. Health care organizations still will tend to receive more payment if they provide more, or more intensive, services to a larger number of persons. They will not be able to dictate what they are paid through their own charge schedules or cost figures, however.

MARKET-BASED DEVELOPMENT

The marketing approach to health services development differs sharply from conventional health system practices. It starts from some notion as to what individuals *need* but goes on to ask how many of them will demand how much from whom and be able to pay how much for it. It is an entirely amoral discipline, though it can be used morally by moral organizations. Using marketing analysis, it still is possible for a health care organization to decide it will offer a service because it's needed, even if the service can't pay for itself. It should enable that organization, however, to make such a decision in an informed, rational manner, fully realizing how many persons will use it and how much of a loss is likely to result.

Marketing can be used to "pander" to the whims of consumer markets, to give them what they want whether or not it's good for them. Such an application clearly is antithetical to the paternal mission of the health care delivery system. On the other hand, marketing also can be used to determine under what circumstances individuals probably will behave the way you'd like them to and use the services you're convinced they need. If you find it feasible and acceptable for you to arrange those circumstances, you can claim legitimately that you are responding to community health needs while, you hope, surviving through the slings and arrows of increasing government regulation.

COMPETITION

Market positioning can be carried out only in relation to the competition. The most effective market position for your organization is where you provide the services you're best qualified to offer (in comparison to others who do or could offer similar services) to persons who will use a sufficient amount of those services to make your program a success (in spite of other things they could do with their time and/or money). Marketing insists that you view yourself from the market's perspective as one of a number of competing choices, and decide where you fit best.

The combination of need-based development and cost-based reimbursement has enabled many health care organizations to become overdeveloped and overreimbursed relative both to the competition and to what society is saying it is willing to accept. Had health care organizations been subject to the same market forces as other industries, or even if they consciously had sought their best market positions despite the absence of such forces, current regulatory efforts might never have been necessary. It is late, but even more important now that the health care system devote its attention to identifying and achieving effective and viable market positions.

Competition always has existed in health care delivery and actually has become more intense over the last two decades. More and more organizations have been attracted into health care delivery by the combination of perceived need, public-spirited mission, and excellent financial prospects. Many have failed, but not as many as tend to fail in other industries. Specific sectors of the system used to have well-defined roles complementary to each other. Now hospitals, nursing homes, physicians, and public health departments find themselves increasingly trying to deliver the same kinds of services to the same kinds of persons.

The absence of an accurate understanding of market positioning and competition has led many organizations to develop programs to provide overlapping services to identical populations. It's an old joke among planning agencies to anticipate that if the local population is expected to grow by 50,000 persons in five years, every hospital in town will insist they must be allowed to expand to serve those same 50,000. In competitive marketing, hospitals might dream of achieving a 100 percent share of this new market, but it is to be hoped that they would be more realistic about their prospects. Moreover, they would identify and implement specific strategies to achieve a strong market share rather than merely insist they deserve one.

In a competitive context, it is most appropriate to identify positions that are relatively unfilled. Developing ambulatory care programs in medically underserved areas or developing services unavailable elsewhere are good examples (birth centers, ambulatory surgery). However, it always must be recognized that even in what appear to be empty spaces for services development, competition exists.

In medically underserved areas, people are coping with their health needs somehow. They may be using a pharmacist, nonprofessional alternatives (*curandera* among the Spanish-speaking, for example), or caring for themselves. Each coping mechanism is competition. You must be able to offer residents of such areas significantly better benefits (product) or significantly less cost (out-of-pocket, waiting time) if you expect them to become patients. Home deliveries and conventional hospital obstetric care are competitors for birth centers; doctors' offices or hospital inpatient surgery compete with ambulatory surgery programs.

PSYCHOLOGICAL MARKET POSITION

The actual market position you hold or aspire to is not the same, necessarily, as how you are viewed by your current and potential markets. The image they have of you ideally should be roughly consonant with reality, while ideally both should be consonant with what you think your role and mission are. The view individuals have of your market position often may differ from both what it is and what you'd like, however. Since it is their perception that influences their market choices, you should be especially sensitive to such discrepancies.

The psychological market position you hold may be different for different market segments, or fairly uniform across all. You may be viewed as:

- the high-class hospital where the latest technology is available but people are treated callously
- the butcher shop where only people who can't afford anyplace else have to go
- the one place in town where people really get tender, loving care
- the program where you have to prove you have money before they'll let you in
- the program where they'll take anybody, but only because they've got no choice
- where "those other people" go (Catholics, whites, osteopaths)
- where they keep you waiting all day before you see anyone
- the highest-priced "hotel" in town

To understand your psychological market position, you must be able to view your transactions from the perspective of your market. The market audit is the principal source of information on your position, especially if it extends beyond your current patients, physicians, etc. To change your psychological position probably will require a combination of changing how you behave and what you tell people. Undoubtedly much can be accomplished through promotional efforts, but unless your communications are consistent with your behavior, the efforts may fail. (See Chapter 7.)

Your psychological market position may aid or severely constrain your program development efforts. Should you attempt to develop new services or attract new markets not consistent with your image, you may have great difficulty. The carriage-trade hospital that seeks to serve a low-income neighborhood or the city hospital hoping to attract affluent suburban patients may fail utterly. The local community general hospital may have great difficulty attracting referrals even if it enhances its specialist capabilities. The nursing home attempting to add home health services or the medical program adding mental health care may encounter similar problems.

Psychological market position may be viewed as a constraint on development—the necessity of developing in ways that are consistent with your current position. If necessary or sufficiently desirable, you may choose to alter your image in order to pave the way for the success of an innovative program or service. The one thing you must avoid in making changes is being ignorant of or disregarding your psychological market position. This is equally as true of reducing or eliminating services as it is of adding new ones or expanding.

There may be good reasons for eliminating obstetric or pediatric services, for example, but the result may be a change in your image as a full-service, family-centered hospital. In some cases, dropping obstetric services may result in losses of gynecological surgery admissions as well. Cutting a well-baby clinic may reduce visits by mothers. The full effects of program changes on your actual and psychological market position should be considered in deciding whether and how to make them.

ESTABLISHING A POSITION

There are two steps in effectively establishing the market position you want:

1. identifying the position you want

2. achieving that position, actually and psychologically

The kind of position you identify as your objective should be the total set of objectives established through market audit and analysis. The specific position that is your target should be the best possible fit between your capabilities, strengths (relative to your competition), and the kinds of products/place/prices your market is most interested in and likely to buy from you.

Marketing insists that you start with who the market is and what it most perceives as needed and is likely to purchase. In other words, you first identify how the market is prepared to behave—the transactions in which it would most probably participate—before you consider how you ought to behave. With an appreciation for how the market proposes to behave, you then examine the transactions in which it would be the most appropriate for you to participate. Your examination will take into account what you can do best as you see it, but also what your competition can do and how the markets are likely to choose if given a choice.

Your identification of what kinds of benefits/services your markets are most interested in should be made as objectively as possible. The greatest danger is that you will make the examination blinded or overfocused by what you really want to do. Your feelings about what the market needs may well be your starting point, but only a start. Unless such needs can and will be translated into actual use, they are meaningful philosophically but limited practically.

Predicting market behavior always is tricky, especially relative to products identified only hypothetically. Market research should help you identify the kinds of needs people perceive for themselves, the mix of product/place/price they seem most prepared to seek and capable of purchasing. Mere prediction is not your only choice, of course, since your educational/promotional efforts can enhance the market's perception of needs and interest in specific services. Market positioning first identifies what markets are interested in what transactions, then asks whether they'd be receptive to what you can offer.

Identifying what represents the most appropriate set of services for you to offer also should be done as objectively as possible. The choice should be based on the extent to which you can achieve the maximum kinds of benefits markets are interested in purchasing, and the effects that foreseeable transactions will have on you and your markets. Can you do the most effective job of offering qualities and quantities of care that match preferences of the market? Will your offering have effects on the community of which you'll be proud? Will the types and levels of transactions you can foresee produce acceptable financial and other net effects on your organization?

Just as you examined causes, behavior, and impacts in your audit of current market relationships, you should do so in selecting your optimal market position. Causes include the factors that will motivate people to seek a given service and choose a specific source. Behavior is the types and amounts of specific services you expect would be used if you offered them. Impacts are the effects the behavior of identified market segments will have on individuals' health and your organization's performance. Similarly, you must identify and anticipate environmental developments, competitive strengths, and potential reactions in planning your own actions.

What market segments are likely to be most receptive to what services? What income levels, health insurance coverage, or government program will cover what costs of providing such services? At what levels of production/utilization of services will your costs be what (break-even analysis)? At those costs and expected revenues, what will be the financial effects? What would be the net overall outcome of your offering that service (given expected cost, use, revenue) on your organization and community?

By answering these questions as objectively and rationally as possible, you can make better decisions on specific programs and—putting them all together—on your market position. By identifying and achieving effective market positions, you are determining what kind of organization/program you should be, and can survive and prosper as. Adoption of a marketing approach requires giving up some of your preference for "doing your own thing" since it requires identifying just what "things" markets will support your doing. On the other hand, you gain the advantage of increasing the probability that doing your thing will have the effects you prefer on you and your community.

COMPETITION OR COORDINATION

A unique and challenging choice available to health care organizations in regard to market positioning is the choice of whether to seek your optimal position through competition or cooperation. In most industries, a market position is achieved through a series of evolutionary developments, of trials and errors, winning some and losing some in competition with other organizations in the same business. Health care organizations are permitted, even encouraged, to work with their peers in the development of regionally coordinated systems of health care delivery.

In effect, planning and regulatory agencies have decreed that the market shall not be permitted to reward the victors and punish the misfits in competitive market positioning in the health field. Certificate-of-need laws and compulsory rate setting dictate how large a given organization may become, what services it may offer, and how much it will be reimbursed for doing. Such controls are general rather than specific in most cases, however, and leave a lot of room for choices about exactly who will do exactly what for exactly whom. As long as costs and quality goals are achieved and access is acceptable, it appears to make no great difference how the specifics are worked out.

Clearly, one way to reduce risks regarding what your competitors will do is to come to some agreement with them regarding what you're going to do for whom vs. what their market position will be. Hospitals have undertaken such arrangements for decades, agreeing that one will do obstetrics and the other pediatrics, or one will take care of emergency medical services and the other will have an oncology unit. Health departments, family planning programs, and hospitals have divided up markets through service on planning councils and coordinating committees.

For a brief period, 1964-66, the Hill-Harris amendments to the Hill-Burton legislation actually provided federal support for such coordinated development efforts. Areawide health facilities planning councils had been developed as early as the 50s, with hospital representatives voting on who should do what and who should expand or offer new services. Health and welfare planning councils, under sponsorship of United Fund or comparable fund-raising groups, accomplished similar cooperative efforts among other health organizations. The antitrust implications of such coordination have yet to be clarified by the judicial system, although a case [1] is under way.

Pending resolution of the legal implications, the choice of competition vs. coordination is up to each health care organization. A preference for coordination by no means eliminates the necessity or value of marketing, however. Having identified what services you intend to provide to what markets, even

---

[1] Hospital Bldg. Co. vs. Rex Hospital Trustees. 425 US 738, 48 L.Ed.2d 338, 96 S. Ct. 1848.

if the competition fully agrees with your position and will avoid duplicating your offering, you still have to get the market to behave as you wish. This means designing and implementing programs whose product/price/place will meet market expectations even if you have no apparent competition. It will place greater emphasis on promotion, on communicating to markets that yours truly is the only game in town.

Coordination of programs is not simply a matter of agreeing to carve up the market. One of the inevitable consequences of such an approach will be the specialization of individual organizations. Rather than trying to do everything for a few, each organization in a regional system will be doing some things for everybody. This will place much emphasis on coordination of programs, services, and information to avoid the fragmentation and discontinuity of care that might result otherwise. It will require that you concentrate some of your marketing effort on another market: your peers in a regionally coordinated system. It will be important for you to understand, predict, and influence their behavior, much as you do for the behavior of physicians and patients. The rules of the game are the same.

SUMMARY

Market positioning probably is the most important concept in marketing. It comprises what you are and to whom, the mix of services you offer (product/place/price), and the people who use them (markets). It covers both what is true as you see it and what the markets perceive to be true. It arises from identifying and merging what people are interested in getting (not merely need) and what you are best qualified to offer (not merely what you'd like to do). It requires asking questions about the market rather than making arbitrary decisions about how individuals should behave. It attempts the most effective, efficient confluence of how the market behaves and how your organization behaves.

Because of the lack of natural market mechanisms, many health care organizations have been free to dictate what they will offer and yet survive even if few markets use them. This unnatural situation is ending. As a result, you will benefit from being able to identify and achieve positions in the market where you can survive and prosper, rather than be guaranteed perpetuity. Your organizations must become more effectively specialized, more sensitive to what the competition is and is capable of doing well. You have to identify and demonstrate what you can do better from the market's perspective.

The psychological side of market positioning involves knowing first how you are perceived. Then you compare it to the "truth" and how you'd like to be perceived, and respond accordingly. While market perceptions may be inaccurate, they have a lot to do with what behavior, what offerings on your part, will be successful. Your image may affect how people behave with respect to you, hence it should be a matter of concern.

To establish and maintain a viable market position, it is necessary that you first understand and predict market behavior. Whatever needs you identify should be capable of becoming effective demands for and use of specific services. You then have to choose which of all possible market behaviors you can most effectively relate to and the services you're most interested in and best qualified to offer. This requires precise identification of the product/place/price mix that will attract sufficient numbers of consumers to make your offering it worthwhile, both to the market and to you.

The unique choice available to health care organizations is that of identifying and achieving optimum market positions through competition or coordination. A position can be established only in relation to both the market and the competition, so you may, in effect, work with your peers to determine what each of you does best. Such a conspiracy would be illegal in most industries and may be so determined in health. The advantages, however, are such that planning and regulatory agencies are promoting and supporting joint or shared planning efforts.

Readings

General

Coleman, J., et al. "A Survey of Financial Planning Models for Health Care Organizations." *Journal of Medical Systems* 2:1, 1978, p. 59.

Cunningham, R. "Face Fewer Admissions, Shorter Stays." *Modern Healthcare*, June 1977, p. 29.

Doherty, N., and Hicks, B. "Cost-Effectiveness Analysis and Alternative Health Care Programs for the Elderly." *Health Services Research* 12:2, Summer 1977, p. 190.

Falberg, W., and Bonnem, S. "Good Marketing Helps a Hospital Grow." *Hospitals, JAHA,* June 1, 1977, p. 70.

Glick, J. "The Hospital: How Will It Survive?" *Hospital Financial Management,* January 1979, p. 12.

Mc Daniel, J. "We Have Seen Rate Review and It Works." *Hospitals, JAHA* 52:8, April 16, 1978, p. 71.

McLaren, J. and Trager, B. "Marketing Assures a Satellite Facility a Safe Send-off." *Hospitals, JAHA,* June 1, 1977, p. 67.

Ross, D., and Tripoli, F. "Fiscal Risks, Methods, Rewards Shape Community Outreach Success." *Hospitals, JAHA,* July 16, 1977, p. 86.

Sacks, T. "It Takes a Sense of Survival." *Hospitals, JAHA,* April 16, 1978, p. 101.

Seaver, D. "Hospital Revises Role, Reaches Out to Cultivate and Capture Markets." *Hospitals, JAHA,* June 1, 1977, p. 59.

Slom, S. "Ghetto Medicine." *The Wall Street Journal,* 58:1, October 21, 1977, p. 1.

Antitrust

Holcomb, B. "Virginia Agency Seeks Antitrust Ruling." *Health Care Week,* 2:1, September 25, 1978, p. 1.

Sellers, B. (ed.). *Antitrust and Health Services: A Second Look* (New York: National Health Council, 1978).

Thompson, M. *Antitrust and the Health Care Provider* (Germantown, Md.: Aspen Systems Corp., 1979).

Chapter 10

Resource Decisions

Among the most important marketing decisions are those related to how many resources would or will be required to carry out a program. Such resources include whatever facilities, personnel, equipment, supplies, and money will be necessary to undertake the behavior you intend. While a full discussion of the subject would take a book by itself,[1] this chapter focuses on how marketing analysis should be incorporated in such a decision.

Two examples of resources are provided: hospitals and primary care programs. Both include facilities as a major resource requirement, although personnel is the main focus for primary care. Personnel is equally as critical as hospital facilities, though regulatory planning requires that the need for facilities be established first. Such an approach for primary care would be totally counterproductive.

While other types of health resources are equally important, it is hoped that these two examples will provide a general approach and a clear illustration of where marketing fits.

HOSPITAL RESOURCES

Market Identification

The first task in preparing for a resource decision is to identify the market, the set of persons who now, or potentially might, use the service you require resources to provide. Separate service markets should be identified for each service you're planning, reflecting realities of the different capacities and attraction power of different services. Burn units could serve an entire state or

---

[1] It has. See the author's *Determining Health Needs,* Ann Arbor, Mich.: Health Administration Press, 1978.

multistate region, while primary care programs may serve only a neighborhood.

The market you identify should satisfy at least three criteria:

1. It should contain almost everyone who has a significant probability of using the service you're planning and should exclude those who don't.
2. It should comprise geopolitical areas whose populations can be described in terms of demographic characteristics that will affect their need for and use of services.
3. These areas should be such that population forecasts for each are available readily.

Depending on the capacity and attraction power of the service you're planning, the market may be made up of census tracts, zip codes, towns and cities, counties, or larger units. When you reach the point where few if any additional patients can be anticipated, you've gone far enough. The market you've identified does not mean that everyone within it will use your service and no one outside it will. It simply means that you plan intensive analysis of everyone within it to predict and influence their use of the service, while you will simply accept and make a rough guess as to how many persons outside the identified market may become customers.

For example, analysis of current patient origin should reveal which communities are the source of how many patients. Communities that currently do, or in the future might, send you significant numbers of patients (only you can decide what numbers are significant) should be included; those that don't or won't shouldn't be included. The more separate communities you include, the more comprehensive and accurate your analysis can be, but also the more complex, time consuming and expensive.

Market Analysis

Once you have identified your total market, you should divide it into market segments. A market segment is simply a subset of the market that:

- is sufficiently homogeneous so that everyone in it can be treated alike
- is sufficiently different that everyone in it should be treated differently from the rest of the market

You may segment the market according to such factors as:

- place of residence
- age, sex, or other demographic characteristics

- income, health insurance coverage
- health status
- physician identification or referral source

You should divide the market into as many segments as are useful and comfortable to handle. Segments should be exclusive and exhaustive for each use; everyone in the market should be placed in a segment, and no one should be in more than one segment.

For each segment you identify, you should establish two kinds of information. First is their contribution to your current patient load (current market). The numbers of admissions, patient days, outpatient visits, surgeries, etc., from each segment should be determined and the percentage each contributes to the total calculated. Second is your market share for each segment. Of all the admissions, patient days, outpatient visits, surgeries, etc., used by persons in each segment, what portion now chooses you as their source of each service?

The analysis of market segments should be portrayed in a matrix such as shown in Figure 10-1. Such a matrix informs you which segments (neighborhoods, social class, physicians, etc.) are the major sources of your patients and what portion of all their current use of a given service comes to you. The overall matrix describes your patient mix and extent of market penetration. Careful analysis of your patient mix should help you decide whether it is optimal in terms of your capacity, mission, and role. Would you rather serve more self-pay patients, more tertiary care patients, more obstetrics and pediatrics, for example? Market penetration data tells you where you have obvious potential for changing your patient mix or increasing use of your service. Large segments where you have small shares represent significant opportunities, while small segments where you have large shares do not.

Figure 10-1 Matrix for Analyzing Market Segments

Segment	# Admissions to Your Hospital	% of All Your Admissions	# Their Admissions to Any Hospital	% Your Market Share
A	400	20	500	80
B	200	10	800	25
C	600	30	1,200	50
D	300	15	1,000	30
E	500	25	5,000	10
Total	2,000	100	8,500	23.5

You should perform this market segment analysis on as many segments and services as are useful. There is no conventional or useful rule. Obviously, the more analysis you do, the more time and money it takes but the better you will understand your market. The more you know, the more you can use a rifle rather than shotgun approach in predicting and influencing future behavior of the market and use of your services.

The data for your market analysis should come mainly from your own records. They should contain past and present descriptions of who uses your services and how many of them. To discover the characteristics of persons in the same segments who don't use your services, you'll have to look outside your institution, however. Local planning agencies may be the source of patient origin data for all local hospitals. Administration of other hospitals may be willing to share their data with you, if you'll share yours with them.

Community surveys may be carried out as a supplement to or substitute for patient origin data. Such surveys also may provide insights into why people choose one source of care over another. In order to discover as basic an item of information as what proportion of a given segment chooses which sources of care, fairly large samples are needed to produce high accuracy. The basic formula for determining the required sample size is as follows:

$$S = \left(\frac{2\sqrt{(p)(1-p)}}{e} \right)^2$$

where   S = sample size required
p = estimated proportion
e = how accurate you wish to be, expressed as $\pm$e (%)

For example, if you wished to estimate the proportion of the population choosing you as a source of care, and you have no idea what it is, your most conservative guess in terms of sample size is that p = .5 (half the population chooses you). To derive an estimate of the true proportion accurate to within $\pm$5%, sample size would be calculated as:

$$S = \left(\frac{2\sqrt{(.5)(.5)}}{.05} \right)^2 = \left(\frac{1}{.05} \right)^2 = 20_2 = 400$$

The further the proportion p gets from .5, the smaller the sample size—e.g., to estimate with the same accuracy for p of around .1, sample size would be

$$S = \left(\frac{2\sqrt{(.1)(.9)}}{.05} \right)^2 = \left(\frac{.6}{.05} \right)^2 = 12_2 = 144$$

The more accurate you wish to be, the larger the sample size has to be. To calculate the true proportion within plus or minus 1 percent could require a sample as large as:

$$S = \left(\frac{2\sqrt{(.5)(.5)}}{.01} \right)^2 = \left(\frac{1}{.01} \right)^2 = 100^2 = 10,000$$

For proportions where you really have no good estimate beforehand, sample sizes required for different accuracy levels would be as follows:

$\pm 10\%$	100
$\pm 5\%$	400
$\pm 2\%$	2,500
$\pm 1\%$	10,000

This sample size requirement is complicated when you're trying to estimate such factors as hospital admissions. Since only about one-eighth of the population is hospitalized in any given year, you would have to survey 800 persons just to get a sample of 100 admissions. For physician visits that are much more common, this is not much of a problem. For emergency rooms, only about 20 percent of the population visits one in a given year; a sample of 500 persons would be required to get 100 who used one.

Once current markets and market shares have been determined, the hospital has the choice of attempting merely to forecast future reality or to influence it. A forecast probably should be done first so the hospital can see whether there is any reason to try to intervene toward influencing the future. If the forecast reveals an optimal patient mix and level of utilization for a given service, with no intervention anticipated, then probably no intervention is appropriate. If the forecast suggests a disaster—low utilization against high fixed costs producing severe losses—some action may seem desirable.

Whatever action is considered, it should be evaluated in terms of its future impact. Actions of closing units or discontinuing money-losing services should be appraised in terms of their overall impact on the community, the hospital's financial position, physicians' attitudes, employee morale, etc. Actions of attempting to increase utilization of services should be evaluated in terms of their costs as well as potential success, in terms of all their impacts on the hospital and community.

Forecasting Utilization

The future utilization of any service the hospital provides is a function of three factors:

1. the future use rate by the market of that particular service in general
2. the size of the population included in the market
3. the proportion of that population that chooses your hospital as the source of that service

If you have identified appropriate markets and segments, the size of the future market population should be known to you through reliable population projections. Having examined current markets and market shares, you will have assessed whether merely to forecast or to attempt to change them. Your final decision should rest on what the overall future utilization will be, and therefore what the use rate by the overall market population will be.

Current population use rates may be hard to calculate unless accurate patient origin and characteristics data are available for your market area. Chances are what data are available will enable you to calculate population use rates only by residence rather than by other segment characteristics. Patient origin data by residence enable you to determine use rates as well as major markets and market shares. If a sample indicates that your hospital gets 20 percent of the annual admissions by a given area (market share) and that you had 200 admissions from that area, then the total admissions would have been 1,000 (200 ÷ 20%). Once you know the population of the area (e.g., 8,000), then you can calculate the admission rate for the population as 1,000 ÷ 8,000 = 125 admissions per thousand per year.

For each segment of your market for which you can identify a current use rate, you should examine whether that rate is likely to change in the future. Just as with market shares and current markets, you have the choice of merely forecasting future use rates or of trying to influence them. Where you feel use rates are low (e.g., for preventive services) you may want to raise them through community education programs or making them more accessible. This may affect both the overall use rate and your market share. Where you feel use rates are too high, you may attempt to reduce them (e.g., second surgical opinions for too much surgery, developing a primary care program to reduce misuse of the emergency room).

Where you hope to change overall use rates, rather than your share of current rates, you should be realistically conservative. Human behavior is hard to change, whether your focus is on physicians or patients. Changes are likely to occur slowly, if they occur at all. In order to change behavior, you should be confident that you understand why people use services at the rate they do now, and convinced that you can so change the incentives that motivate their behavior that they will respond in the direction you prefer and predict.

Forecasting Methods

For the service use rates to be forecast for each market population, there are a number of technical, quantitative methods available. Each requires identifying past use rates as a basis for calculating and projecting trends into the future. One way is to identify factors associated with past trends so that future developments in such factors (age, sex, income, morbidity) can be used as a basis for predicting future use rates. Regardless of the technique used, unless the reasons for past trends are known and their continuing impact confidently anticipated, it makes no particular sense to project past trends mechanically into the future.

Measures of the accuracy of forecasting methods such as simple and multiple regressions describe only how close they came to estimating past values. Assuming such accuracy for their projections of the future is no more than a convenient assumption. In numerous cases, past trends will project no use for some services, or doubling every year or so, neither of which may be truly probable in fact even if mathematically justified in theory.

Some complex formulas may be useful as simulations to predict what would happen if a specific factor were changed deliberately (supply of physicians, charges, etc.). In such cases, both the accuracy of the entire formula and the reliability of the specific factor have to be examined carefully. No forecast or simulation can be anything more than an intelligent guess about the future. It is wiser to identify factors that are likely to change and whose impact on use rates is understood as a basis for predicting the future than it is to accept a mathematical projection without thinking.

Because forecasts are (one hopes) educated guesses, care must be taken whenever a decision is based on one. Where a forecast anticipates substantial changes in use rates in future years, a substantial change may be required. Common sense suggests delaying the change, where possible, to see if it begins or continues to happen as anticipated, rather than to jump in with both feet. Making too many resources available on the basis of forecast increases that don't occur will result in unused capacity, high costs, etc. Making too few because declines in utilization were projected incorrectly will deprive individuals of care, will anger physicians, etc. Given the relative permanence of resources once they're developed, and the difficulty of making fine-tuning adjustments in resources in a short time, forecasting is a headache.

Forecasting Results

Since it is use rates of a service by a population that are forecast, the level of future utilization you expect must be calculated based on the anticipated population. Since forecasting population levels and characteristics also involves uncertainties, your forecast of future utilization is doubly hazardous. Such uncertainties are unavoidable in the nature of forecasting. All that can be suggested is that care be taken in basing decisions on forecasts.

One useful approach to evaluating how dangerous forecasting errors might be is called *sensitivity analysis.* This kind of analysis seeks to predict what you feel are the probable ranges of future utilization levels, highest to lowest, and what difference these make to your decision. For example, if you were confident future use rates for medical-surgical care would be between 750 and 850 patient days per thousand, and that future population would be between 200,000 and 220,000, then future utilization should fall between extremes of $200,000 \times 750/1,000 = 150,000$ and $220,000 \times 850/1,000 = 187,000$ patient days. If you feel your share of that utilization will be between 15 and 20 percent, then your utilization should be between $.15 \times 150,000 = 22,500$ and $187,000 \times .20 = 37,400$ patient days.

Because of these areas of uncertainty, the resulting range is substantial. To perform a sensitivity analysis, you must determine how your decision would be affected if future use turns out to be 22,500 patient days vs. 37,400 patient days. If you know you must have 30,000 patient days to justify a decision (e.g., break-even point), then this range might be fine, since the necessary level falls in the middle. If you needed 35,000 patient days, however, you would be much less confident. One or more of the factors would have to end up at the high end of its expected range, and all three probably would have to be above the average.

Since you can influence at least one of the factors (market share), you may be willing to gamble on getting 35,000 patient days. If you can delay your decision, of course, you can wait to see if future developments conform to the trend you projected before making a commitment. By identifying the point(s) at which a different resource decision would result (e.g., buy or lease, build or not, eliminate service or not), you can make better use of the uncertain forecasts you have available.

The resultant forecast should be expressed as the number of units of service you expect in some future year (admissions, average length of stay, physician visits, number of services per visit, x-rays, lab tests, etc.). For inpatient care, total patient days should be calculated together with average daily census (annual patient days ÷ 365). Separate projections should be made for each separate service you're planning.

Resource Requirements

Determining optimal resources for a given level of utilization is a decision based on what you consider to be optimal performance for those resources. No single technique is available for making such a determination. The number of beds per service, physicians per department, size of units, and location of resources all impact on performance in complex ways. Cost, quality, access, and satisfaction all are important performance factors to consider. Selecting an optimal resource alternative, even if future utilization were known perfectly, is a complex decision where no simplistic formula can do.

The most sensible way to choose the optimal resource decision, once a utilization level (or range) has been forecast, is to select what promises the best overall performance. Greater access (ability to accommodate the level and variations in demand) can be purchased only at the risk of increasing costs. Cost savings may require compromises on quality, satisfaction, and access. No single best performance mix can be identified. You must decide what performance factors to consider, predict the impact alternative resource decisions would have on each, and choose what promises the best mix.

Performance factors worth considering should be made operational and described in quantitative terms wherever possible. Costs can be expressed in costs per patient day, unit of service, or episode of care. The costs of maintaining empty beds or constructing new ones should be estimated specifically. Revenue as well as expenditures, and net operating gain or loss, should be projected for each decision based on the projected utilization and reimbursement levels. Occupancy of acute or long-term care beds at best are indirect measures of efficiency and nowhere near as useful as specific cost data in making decisions.

Quality should be considered and examined in specific, quantitative terms as well, if possible. A number of quality-related standards may be employed—minimum utilization levels for sophisticated, expensive services such as megavoltage radiation therapy (300 cases per year), open-heart surgery (200 procedures per year), etc. Minimum sizes for specific services may be adopted as standards (20 beds for pediatric units, 15 beds for neonatal intensive care units (ICUs)). Where possible, direct measures such as mortality, complication rates, etc., should be used rather than relying on indirect indicators.

Access may be examined in a number of contexts. The actual time it takes your patients to reach the source of your services, to get an appointment, be admitted, or be seen all are access measures. So is the extent to which your charges, impersonal treatment of patients, hours of operation, etc., act as barriers to use by specific segments. One useful and fairly precise measure of access is the probability that a patient can be accommodated in the appropriate unit when an admission is requested.

Demand for inpatient care varies substantially over time (day of the week, time of the year, holiday or vacation, etc.). Demand for outpatient services also will vary, by all of those factors and by time of the day as well. Ability to accommodate such variations is a specific measure of access likely to be reflected in satisfaction levels of patients and physicians. Such variations can be predicted with fair accuracy—at least the extent of variations, if not their timing.

Given the reality of varying demand, you have two basic choices in your resource decisions. First, you can attempt to gear your operational capacity to conform to variations in demand. This can be done through temporary employment, on-call part-time help, etc. Given the high fixed costs of most services, substantial negative impacts on cost/efficiency still will result when utilization varies greatly. The other choice is to attempt to control variations in demand via appointment systems, admissions scheduling, etc. Such devices can improve the cost/efficiency of high fixed-cost services such as inpatient care, provided physicians and patients are willing to accept controls on their behavior.

Daily variations in hospital census, for specific services (medical-surgical, obstetric, pediatric, psychiatric, etc.) and for the hospital as a whole, can be predicted with substantial accuracy. For most small units, where average daily census is 20 or less, daily variations conform to the Poisson, a common statistical distribution model. Consulting a Poisson table, available in most statistics texts, will inform decision makers how often specific census levels above the mean are likely to occur. For a unit with an average census of two, for example, census levels of eight or more will occur only .1 percent of the time, roughly once every two years. Census levels of seven or higher are likely only .3 percent of the time, or once a year, etc.

For psychiatric and rehabilitation units of any size, and for other services with average census of higher than 20, a Normal distribution model provides slightly better estimates of high census levels. Once the mean (average daily census) and standard deviation of the census distribution are estimated, the frequency of any census level above the mean can be estimated. Because of the extreme low census levels that occur during the Christmas, New Year's and other holiday periods, census levels below the mean don't fit the model as well.

The Normal distribution is such that census levels 3 standard deviations or more above the mean will only occur .13 percent of the time, or once every two years, 2.33 standard deviations or more only 1 percent of the time, 1.96 standard deviations or more 2.5 percent, and 1.65 or more 5 percent of the time. With the aid of the Poisson and Normal distributions, it is possible to determine how frequently a given bed supply would tend to be exceeded, hence you could determine what bed supply is necessary to accommodate demand what percent of the time.

When demand tends to exceed bed supply, hospitals have a number of choices, of course. If the supply of beds in one service is inadequate, excess patients may be placed in another service. If this is inappropriate or impossible, patients may be placed, perhaps temporarily, in a hall bed, doubling up beds in private rooms, etc. In other circumstances, admissions may be delayed, or referred to another hospital. Deciding the optimal bed supply will reflect how much inconvenience the hospital is willing to endure (or have its patients endure) plus how much it feels is appropriate to spend in extra costs for rarely used capacity to avoid such inconvenience.

For a hospital with an average census of 25 and a standard deviation of 6, it would require six beds to reduce the occurrence of inconvenience from 2.5 percent of the time (eight days a year) to .1 percent of the time (one day every two years). For a hospital with an average daily census of 250 and a standard deviation of 21, it would cost 21 beds to achieve the same reduction in inconvenience. Each institution has to decide (and perhaps convince regulatory agencies) how much it is willing to spend to reduce inconvenience, or how much inconvenience it is willing to endure in order to improve efficiency.

There is no single rule that can or should be followed in all cases. Not only the frequency but also the seriousness of running out of beds has to be considered. Obstetric, psychiatric, and coronary care patients rarely can have their admissions delayed or be adequately cared for in another unit. Where a hospital is the only one available in 50, 100, or more miles, it may be considered necessary to maintain sufficient beds for any contingency. (A supply 4 standard deviations above the mean would be adequate all but one day every 91 years).

All that is necessary to incorporate ability to accommodate varying census levels in resource decisions is to estimate the mean and standard deviation of the census for each service, and for the hospital as a whole. Conventional assumptions have held that the standard deviation is equal to the square root of the mean (average daily census—ADC). This is simply not true. Different services have different standard deviations at the same average census levels. As census levels get larger, the standard deviation becomes increasingly greater than the square root of ADC.

Based on studies of hospitals in five states covering 125 hospital/years of daily census data, the following formula provides accurate working estimates of the standard deviation above the mean once the average daily census has been forecast.

$$S.D. = ADC^{.545}$$

where

S.D. = standard deviation

ADC = projected average daily census

Three factors contribute significantly to differences in census variation. Census levels in larger units or hospitals vary more than smaller, but only relatively so. (Peak census in a 25-ADC facility might be 72 percent above the mean, while in a 250-ADC hospital, the same peak would be only 25 percent above the mean.) Variability in units with longer length of stay (psychiatric, rehabilitation, alcohol treatment, etc.) is less than that in units with shorter stays. In units where a larger proportion of admissions is schedulable (pediatrics, surgery), variation tends to be greater than in units where fewer admissions can be scheduled (obstetrics, psychiatric).

The fact that scheduled services tend to experience more variation in census than those less subject to scheduling indicates that most scheduling is done to serve the convenience of patients and physicians rather than to attain optimum efficiency. Conscious efforts to control scheduling of elective admissions could reduce variations in census significantly, avoiding extreme low and high periods. Such controls could enhance quality and reduce costs by enabling hospitals to maintain appropriate staffing ratios. Where the necessity of additional capital expenditures for expanded or renovated capacity can be avoided through admissions scheduling, even greater benefits can be achieved.

Decisions as to whether to offer a given service should be made in recognition of the added quality or improved access to care such a decision would yield, relative to its cost. If other hospitals provide the same service already, can you really do it better? Is that the best bargain you can make for what it will cost? Given the emphasis on cost containment and threats of increasing regulation of hospitals and other health care delivery organizations, any new service or increase in capacity has to be reviewed skeptically. Where such changes can be justified in terms of significant improvement in service to the community, they should be pursued; where not, they should be avoided. The planning process described here should assist in both deciding and justifying any proposed change.

AMBULATORY-PRIMARY CARE RESOURCES

The specific unit of resource in the production of primary care and most other ambulatory care (exceptions being ambulatory surgery and kidney dialysis) is the professional. Whether physician, physician's assistant, nurse practitioner, or other professional, it is the person, not the building, that is the principal resource necessary. To plan for primary care resources is to decide how many persons are required to provide the amounts and types of services to be used by the population to be served.

The traditional model still holds: (1) identifying the community to be served, then (2) basing utilization projections on the synthesis of how they should and do use health services, then (3) deciding on resources needed to provide such services. The third step, however, has to be split into two parts: deciding how many of what types of professionals are required to provide the services, then determining how many of what kinds of facilities are needed to accommodate such professionals and their patients. Both resource decisions will be based on whatever is determined to be the best possible (optimal) performance that can be achieved.

Market Identification

The first task in determining ambulatory-primary care needs is the identification of the community whose need for primary care is the basis for your planning effort. If you break down primary services into pediatric, obstetric/gynecological, medical, mental health, dental, ocular, etc., you should break down the population served accordingly. Pediatric services apply only to children, obstetrics/gynecology only to women, and so on.

Primary care planning areas should be designated as a starting point for identifying the community. Such areas should be designed to circumscribe populations who would be within acceptable travel time/distance from a source of primary care if there were one central to the area. This is a purely hypothetical area in that persons within it will not necessarily use the resources located there. However, it will serve to identify areas where, if there are no primary resources at all, there probably are individuals who have access problems.

The areas and resident populations thus identified should be such that future population and demographic characteristic estimates can be obtained for them. Such data are useful, if not essential, in determining their future need for and use of primary health services. Data on their actual behavior— current use of primary care services, choice of sources, etc.—may be difficult to come by, but would be worth estimating from sample surveys.

Within each primary care planning area, the first issue is whether or not a source of primary care exists (is available) at all. Second is the question of whether a sufficient number of providers will exist to handle the volume of primary care use that should and will occur in the future. To make such a judgment, two data items are necessary:

1. how many units of service (e.g., primary care visits) will be appropriately demanded in the future
2. what amount of services the average provider (physician, other) can produce annually at optimal cost, quality and access

Future Use

The future use of primary care by a designated community is a function of two factors:

1. the use rate (visits per person per year) by that population
2. the size of the population

Use rates that will occur in the future are a synthesis of what professionals think individuals should use (need) and what the community actually tends to use (demand). If you believe persons in a community should use more or less primary care (e.g., preventive services), then you may choose to set targets and determine strategies for achieving changes in behavior. Among such strategies are those involving making sources of care more accessible or acceptable, such as by adding some to the current supply, changing health insurance coverage, enhancing competition, and so on.

Some predictable developments no doubt will affect future use of primary care without your intervention: changes in education levels, income or health insurance benefits, age groups, disease patterns, national health insurance, HMO growth, etc. All may alter use of primary care, whether or not you approve. Such developments and their impact should be identified and anticipated in estimating as well as targeting future primary care use.

There are essentially two components of use rates for primary care. First is the proportion of the population that will have *any* primary care contacts in a given year. This is largely a function of patient choice as to whether to seek a contact, but certainly is affected by the accessibility of sources for care. Second is the average number of visits per year for the proportion of persons who make visits. This is more a function of provider choice in recommending additional visits, although the consumer also has a say in it.

This two-part breakdown corresponds roughly to admission rate and length of stay for inpatient services. By multiplying the two, an overall use rate of average visits per person per year is calculated. It is important to know this and it is a distinction worth retaining as to the two components that make up this use rate. Trends, developments, and strategies may affect each differently. Only by addressing them separately can you develop accurate estimates of future use.

Where you determine changes in use are desirable, you should identify intervention strategies. Future use patterns then will be based on how successful you expect your strategies to be. Since the use of primary care is likely to be more optional and more subject to consumer choice, both forecasting and achieving changes in individual behavior are likely to be difficult. The effects of changes in the use of primary care on the use of other services (inpatient care) should be anticipated specifically and carefully.

The same methods used for forecasting inpatient use are available for primary care. Demographic changes are likely to influence both the number and type (initial vs. follow-up, acute vs. chronic) of primary care used. These changes may be identified through factor forecasting or trend analysis. Expert panels may provide useful insights into both primary care use problems and potential interventions. Any forecast necessarily is a guess, of course, and should be treated gingerly. A range of visits probably would be a more realistic forecast than a precise number.

Resource Requirements

The first resource required for primary care delivery is the person, the specific health care professional who will provide the care. How many providers are required depends on how many units of service (visits) each can be expected to make within acceptable or desirable limits of cost, quality, and access. It may be that a family practitioner can provide 10,000 inexpensive visits per year, but only by using assembly line techniques involving dubious quality and long waits. On the other hand, a provider might be able to offer ideal quality and immediate access with an average of 2,000 visits per year, but the cost would be exorbitant.

The cost of primary care reflects not simply expenses to the provider, but how much providers choose to charge. The productivity and quality of the provider reflects training, attitudes, and willingness to work some number of hours per week. Access is affected by provider willingness to function on evenings and weekends, as well as choice of practice site. Rarely can such choices be regulated externally, though some incentives are available to make one choice more attractive than another to a physician (e.g., subsidized practice).

Productivity of physicians is difficult to predict, since each can decide to alter productivity from one day to the next. Some rough estimates can be gained from American Medical Association reports on average productivity for different categories of practitioners: G.P.s, F.P.s, pediatricians, obstetricians, internists, etc. Each tends to have a slightly different average productivity based on solo vs. group practice, number of hours per week, age, and so forth.

Productivity of physicians is something that can be targeted for change (as with census variability in inpatient units) rather than merely predicted. Promoting growth of HMOs or group vs. solo practice, augmenting the supply of physician extenders as assistants to or even surrogates for physicians in some cases, can have deliberate consequences on productivity. Just as use patterns should be predicted based on intervention strategies, so should productivity levels.

Once productivity rates (visits per practitioner per year) have been forecast, the number of practitioners required can be calculated. If a population is expected to use 60,000 primary care visits per year, and each physician provider is expected to handle 6,000, then the need for practitioners is $60,000 \div 6,000 = 10$.

The need for facilities to provide ambulatory/primary care is another matter. Depending on the situation, actual or desirable accommodations may be private physicians' offices, group practice clinics, public health department clinics, or hospital outpatient departments. Each is so different that no direct estimation of ambulatory facility requirements is possible even after the number of physicians required has been determined. Each primary care planning area should be examined individually to determine what facility is appropriate.

In many such areas, a sufficient supply or perhaps even a surplus of providers may be apparent. In others, a severe shortage may appear. A first requirement in assessing such situations is to determine whether contiguous areas serve each other. Where one area with a surplus of providers is adjacent or very near to another with no providers or a severe shortage, individuals may be able to travel from the shortage area to a surplus region with no ill effects. Unless community surveys reveal significant dissatisfaction with such travel, no attempt to relocate providers may be necessary or even desirable.

Where a shortage exists and is not mitigated or eliminated by a nearby source of care, however, the facility may be viewed as part of a strategy for change. In some such cases, the public health department may be the only potential provider interested in offering service to an underserved population. In others, a special federal or foundation grant (Health in Underserved Rural Areas—HURA—or Robert Wood Johnson Foundation) may attract a hospital or other large organization to offer primary care. In still others, private practitioners may be recruited through community efforts, developmental support, etc.

Facility requirements can be determined only on the type of provider (pediatrician vs. obstetrician vs. family practitioner), anticipated productivity levels, and the type of organization that will sponsor or house the provider. Public health departments may wish different types, amounts, and sizes of treatment, examining, and waiting rooms than do hospitals or medical groups. Private practitioners will make up their own minds and presumably develop their own accommodations without help or control from the planning agency.

The number of rooms required should be determined based on the ability of each room to accommodate the way the provider will practice and the patient use the services. Where a provider uses bloc appointments or accepts walk-ins only, a large waiting area may be necessary. Where physicians use many assistants, many more rooms per visit may be needed than if they work alone. Where the provider functions 12 hours a day, seven days a week, each room can accommodate more patients than where it is used only four hours a day, three days a week.

The basic items needed to calculate room requirements involve the following:

1. number of patients expected per average day
2. peak day patient loads, how large, and how frequent
3. number of hours facility will accommodate patients
4. number of patients per hour each room can handle
5. number of days per week and weeks per year facility is open

These items are combined in this calculation:

hours per day $\times$ visits per room per hour = visits accommodated per room per day

    average or peak load per day divided by visits accommodated per day = number of rooms required to accommodate average or peak load.

The tyranny of averages may be a problem in this calculation. If, in some weeks, productivity is down to fewer visits accommodated per day, or if productivity is less on some days than others, the performance of the provider and the facility may falter. Longer waits than expected will result unless visit volumes drop commensurately. How often peak visit loads will occur and how high they get compared to average productivity also will have a significant effect on waiting time for appointment, waits to be seen, etc.

Like any other resource, the right or best primary care resource configuration is the one that promises and eventually delivers the best mix of performance: cost, quality, and access. Measuring this performance, and forecasting it in advance in order to make resource decisions, is no easy matter, however. Cost may be estimated as charges per visit, but also may include cost to the patient due to hours of operation (having to take off from work or school) lost time and wages due to waiting for an appointment, or even to be seen once having arrived at the facility. Both the facility and the individual provider's behavior affect such costs.

Quality presumably is reflected in the amount of time the provider spends with the patient, but also by a host of other factors not so easily measurable. The qualifications of the provider (general vs. family practitioner, M.D. vs. assistant, specialist vs. generalist, board eligible vs. certified, etc.) all may affect quality. So, too, the personal choice of the provider and other professionals will affect quality more than sheer numbers of providers or facilities.

Even access is a complex factor. Time/distance of travel is covered by design of the service planning areas. Other measures of access include the cost to the patient of care, how the patient is received by the provider, procedures for registration, etc. Length of time to get an appointment, length of wait to be seen, and delays waiting for test results all affect the price a patient pays for care, how long a period must be spent receiving it, and the likelihood that appropriate follow-up visits will be made.

The best you can do is address the performance factors you feel are important, and those on which you reasonably can estimate the effects of resource decisions. You never will be sure the resources will behave exactly as you'd anticipated, but you should estimate their performance and make decisions accordingly.

Chapter 11

Marketing Management

Most health care organizations are staffed and manned without marketing programs and personnel. To implement a marketing program, regardless of scope, it will be necessary to identify or recruit, organize, and manage the resources required to carry it out. Just as the resources for a service program should be based on performance desired and expected, so should the resources necessary to implement marketing efforts. The costs vs. benefits of specific amounts, types, and organizations for such resources also must be evaluated.

There are five major components of the organization that should be considered in managing a marketing program:

1. the governance function: administration-medical staff-governing board/ owner/accountable public body
2. program management and labor, the persons who deliver your services
3. the development or fund-raising function
4. public or community relations, the communications function
5. the planning function, whether short- or long-range

GOVERNANCE

Marketing is far too important a function to be left to a purely staff person or department. At least eventually, those involved in the governance of the organization must be involved in marketing also. To be most effective, a marketing effort must include sensitivity on the part of owners, governing bodies, and accountable public bodies to its policy and financial implications. Medical staff involved in program development also must be aware of the marketing program and sensitive to how their actions and decisions affect market relations. Administrative staff members also must participate in market analysis, strategy development, implementation, and evaluation, and be equally aware of how their behavior affects market relationships.

Governing bodies or community advisory boards may provide direct assistance to a marketing effort. By recruiting members who have marketing, research, and advertising backgrounds, the organization can benefit from free expert advice. Community advisory boards may provide market audit insights into community attitudes, perceived needs, problems, threats, and opportunities. Specific members may have insights into market segments and provide useful advice on promotional efforts directed at those segments. Boards, auxiliaries, and volunteers may be effective promoters of your programs among their acquaintances, adding to your word-of-mouth advertising.

Ideally, marketing should be carried out at the governance level as a distinct function of administration. In smaller organizations, this means the administrator should take on the responsibility; in larger institutions, one of the administrative staff members, preferably the No. 2 or No. 3 person, no lower. In a multiinstitution chain or integrated system, a director of marketing may be employed, though at a level where overall management decisions are made rather than as a staff support function. The information generated through the market audit and market research will reflect the entire organization's program; decisions on marketing strategy will involve the entire institution. Marketing, to be optimally effective, should be endorsed and assimilated as a philosophy of management and performance by the entire organization.

For large organizations such as hospitals, a committee approach may be useful in introducing or even in the long-range conduct of a marketing program. Where power to affect the organization's programs is distributed widely, the committee may be the only practical mechanism for involving and protecting divergent interests. Staff support for the committee should be a specific and important assignment for administration, which certainly will be represented on the committee itself. In addition to standing committees, similarly representative task forces may be used for specific program decisions. In all such cases, representation of the marketing panel should prove a useful addition to members from internal groups: medical staff, board, nursing, administration, and ancillary services.

Involving owners, administrators, medical staff, and board members in most organizations will be a challenge where marketing is an unfamiliar philosophy. For public health care organizations, the involvement of politically responsible officials may prove even more difficult. There may be exaggerated sensitivity among publicly funded health care programs to both the label and the philosophy of marketing. To the extent that marketing can identify more accurately the markets for public services and factors affecting their use and acceptance, it should be appropriate. Where changing the label will decrease sensitivity, this is simple enough.

The hardest point to gain acceptance at the governance level may be the fact that neither marketing nor organizational success are exclusively functions of growth. Increasingly, the challenge to health care organizations will be to get by with fewer resources, to focus program efforts toward greater efficiency rather than expansion. It is unfortunate that there are no positive words for maintaining a healthy situation without growth; all we call it is stagnation. Marketing should increase the viability of your programs and their beneficial impact on the communities you serve, but resource constraints will mitigate against ensuring continued growth even for successful organizations.

PROGRAM MANAGEMENT AND YOUR EMPLOYEES

The total involvement of those who execute your programs is just as critical as that of governance for an effective marketing program. The way your employees, department heads, etc., behave *is,* in effect, your product. Because of the unique, public service, professionally dominated nature of the health care field, administration essentially has less control over that product than in most other industries. Yet since your product is a service, the way your internal staff behaves is most critical.

To be attuned to the marketing program and supportive of it, as well as to appreciate how important their behavior is, your internal staff members should be part of designing, executing, and evaluating the program. They should review the results of the market audit and be helped to understand how their behavior affects its results. They should participate in discussions and the formulation of market goals and objectives if they are expected to help you reach them.

Particularly should they be part of the identification, examination, and evaluation of specific marketing strategies. They eventually must ratify any strategy that requires change in their behavior; if they participate in deciding what change is necessary and why, their implementation of change should be enhanced. Similarly, they should participate in the evaluation of strategies they take part in implementing. Their insights into effects as well as acceptance of evaluation results will be helpful in the evaluation process specifically and management generally.

The mode of their participation will have to be a representative one. Informally, they should be encouraged to participate in t-group or focus group discussions on specific marketing issues and to lend their suggestions to discussions generally. Formally, their representatives should sit on the committees and task forces that design the market audit, evaluate its results, develop goals and objectives, determine strategy, and analyze outcomes. Where market analysis and strategy focuses on specific departments and programs, their representation should increase, even to the point of having all program staff members participate.

The solution to any market problem or the attainment of any market objective can be understood in terms of changing somebody's behavior. The better your staff members understand this principle and can use it in a marketing construct, the more effective your market analysis, strategy, and outcomes will be. By participating in marketing discussions, they will learn a great deal, but so will you. Their insights into why they behave one way, or why consumers do, should prove invaluable to you.

DEVELOPMENT

Not all health organizations have a formal development program or staff, but most have to perform its basic functions: obtaining sufficient funds to operate, replace, or expand capital capacity. Whether this function is carried out through lobbying activities related to public budgets and appropriations, grants from government or foundations, or fund drives in the community, it essentially is a marketing activity in that it attempts to predict and influence behavior. Moreover, its functions are an important part of an overall marketing program.

Some hospital development staff members, or persons with development functions in other organizations, cover a wider range of activities than merely fund raising. They participate in or perhaps lead discussions as to what programs the organizations should develop, as well as where funds might be obtained to provide capital. In effect, they perform much of the marketing function in institutions that have no one else to do it. Whether or not they employ marketing concepts and techniques to do so, in many organizations they are the marketing staff and program.

In institutions that propose to develop an explicit, comprehensive marketing program, the development function and staff will have to be accommodated. Where past involvement has been limited to fund raising, the development staff can be retained in a separate identity, no more subservient to marketing than they are subordinate to overall administration. The marketing program may be able to provide useful information to the development staff on community attributes and attitudes. These should aid fund-raising activities by singling out the most promising market segments from those that need more work.

The development staff also should be able to assist the marketing program by supplying insights on the kinds of sources for capital fund raising that are available, and the potential amounts that might be obtained for specific purposes. In examining the feasibility of alternative market strategies, such information should prove invaluable. The marketing and development staffs should be able to build a symbiotic relationship within the organization where both retain separate identity.

Where the development staff has participated in or actually been responsible for conducting a substantial portion of the marketing function, accommodation may be more of a problem. In some cases, past performance may be reflected by formally designating the development staff as responsible for the marketing program. If the available person or persons have the essential knowledge and skills, or can augment what they have with additional training, this may well work out. There are few professionals available with the health system and marketing training and experience that would be ideal for the marketing program.

If the development staff does take on the marketing function, some adjustments will be necessary. Unless the staff has been part of top-level administration, it should be elevated to that status as part of taking on marketing. Additional staff resources should be assigned to permit adding functions not part of the former development function. Data base and budget capacity will have to be augmented to accommodate the greater responsibilities of a full marketing program.

Where a development function does exist that has performed and appears capable of increasing its marketing contributions, the phasing in of a marketing program is simplified. In keeping with the incremental strategy for introducing the market audit (Chapter 4) and overall marketing (Chapter 12), a preexisting set of related activities may provide a basis for making gradual changes toward a full marketing program. The risk of such a nibbling approach will be that insufficient success will be generated by incidental changes to create the interest in and acceptance of marketing necessary to go the whole way. Where a program has a major identity and responsibility other than marketing, the tendency will be for it to give greater attention to what it more explicitly and obviously is accountable for.

Where a new marketing person is brought in to perform the full marketing function, and the development function has carried out many marketing activities in the past, some conflicts almost inevitably will result. For the marketing program to be most effective, development should be focused specifically on fund raising and capital acquisition rather than program development. This focusing may be viewed as a demotion by the development staff. Whether it would accept the role of continuing to have some marketing responsibilities but under the supervision of a director of marketing will have to be examined in each case.

Where development and marketing are in potential conflict, it should be recognized that marketing is the broader scope, though not necessarily more important, of the two. It is to be hoped that the marketing and development staffs will be able to work out an accommodation regarding who is responsible for what and how related functions will be coordinated. Administration will have to serve as mediator and final judge, including deciding what budget allocations will be made to each and how the performance of each will be evaluated.

Development and marketing always will overlap, though they need not conflict. If the role and responsibilities of each are clarified, and mechanisms for their coordination established and used, they should be mutually supportive. Achieving the necessary clarification and coordination of these functions will require substantial effort as the marketing program is introduced.

PUBLIC RELATIONS

Like development, not all health organizations have a formal public or community relations function, but all perform its basic activities: communication with the wider community about the affairs of the organization. In many organizations, public/community relations may consist of no more than developing and publishing messages to the public regarding what's going on at the institution. Even at this modest level, the function clearly is important to the marketing program, since it would include all promotional activities.

Where public relations is limited to communicating outward from the organization, its accommodation with a marketing program should be fairly simple. Marketing would devise specific messages on the promotion of the organization or its programs and public relations would arrange their dissemination. This could include publicity, advertising, or the combination discussed in Chapter 7. Marketing simply would be one of the groups within the organization that had information to be communicated. The information gained from market audits and market research should help focus and improve public relations efforts. Specific segments, beliefs, and attitudes could be targeted for change and subsequent surveys used to determine whether changes have occurred.

In this simple coexistence, marketing would be very concerned about P.R., since the messages going out from the organization affect its psychological market position as well as the extent to which the public is aware of and possibly interested in the organization's programs. Public relations still could retain a separate identity, however, subject to overall control by administration where marketing would have a major role and influence. Such peaceful coexistence should be sought wherever possible.

In other organizations, public or community relations has expanded its communications function to cover information coming into the organization as well as going out of it. Where this expanded P.R. function exists, it begins to overlap significantly with marketing, specifically duplicating the function of market audit and research. Where the P.R. staff has taken on the added responsibilities of responding to what information it gets from the public (e.g., complaints) and recommending changes in the organization's program, the overlap becomes even greater.

The issue of what to do about such an overlap essentially is similar to that related to development. If the public relations staff can take on the entire marketing function effectively by expanding its knowledge, skills, and resources, this may prove an expedient accommodation. The redesignation of the P.R. function then should be made explicit by changing titles and level in the organization, being sure, however, that marketing doesn't get lost in a purely communications emphasis. As was true for development, designation of the public relations department as responsible for marketing entails the same advantages in an incremental strategy, but also the same risks.

If the overlap is extensive but new staff members are brought in to take on a full marketing program, conflict also is likely to be unavoidable. Because of the scarcity of qualified health/marketing professionals, the marketing staff may well have less background and experience in health than the existing public relations or development staff members already performing many marketing functions.

Here, too, the roles and responsibilities of marketing vs. public relations must be delineated carefully and explicitly. Any redundancy that remains in the two ought to be recognized and accepted only if it is reinforcement rather than duplication, and should be coordinated in any case. The administration again will have to act as mediator and final arbiter to ensure that effective working relationships can be built between the two departments. You'll have to use your own judgment as to the optimal form for such relationships.

The clear distinction between public relations and marketing in general has been that public relations uses communication to change knowledge, beliefs, and attitudes in the community. What and whether behavioral changes result is a matter of independent concern. Marketing employs communication *and performance* to change behavior, in which knowledge, beliefs, and attitudes may be involved. This distinction should provide a basis both for distinguishing and coordinating the two functions. Again, marketing simply is wider in scope, although not necessarily more important, than public relations.

PLANNING

Unlike public relations and development, there isn't a convenient separate existence for planning and marketing. The function of planning is the design and management of change. Unless its function is limited strictly to spatial analysis and architectural planning, the extent of overlap between planning and marketing is likely to be too great for a separate but equal accommodation. Good planning should incorporate marketing concepts and techniques in data gathering, analysis, strategy development, implementation, and evaluation. Marketing does what planning does in health care organizations: it identifies problems, sets goals and objectives, and evaluates strategies and outcomes.

Surprisingly, while development and public relations professionals—especially P.R. professionals—have demonstrated a great deal of interest in marketing, planners have showed little. This may be due to their recognition that marketing is a threat or their feeling that it is a fad that will go away. Neither is a truly good reason for ignoring marketing, however.

Marketing certainly is a potential threat to planning as a profession. If marketing is recognized and incorporated into most health care institutions, there will be little left for planners to do. On the other hand, planners already should possess roughly 80 percent of the knowledge and skills necessary to marketing. By adding marketing concepts and techniques, planners should be able to perform rather than compete with the marketing function in most health organizations. To do so will require accepting the legitimacy and usefulness of marketing and its appropriate incorporation of the planning function.

Planning always has had an image problem since it is an activity rather than a discipline, a function more than a profession. Moreover, planning tends to be relegated to a separate staff function, conducting studies and performing analyses in order to make recommendations to management. Marketing has to be part of management and directly involved in implementation, not just recommendation, and in action, not merely analysis.

The proper role for planners is not to hope marketing is a fad that will go away but to recognize that it contains ways to broaden the scope and increase the effectiveness of the organization's planning and development function. By adding a focus on behavior to its approach and a few market research techniques to its skills, planning should be able to expand to cover marketing in most health organizations. As long as there is a shortage of qualified health marketing professionals, this option represents a viable approach to increasing the role and importance of planning. If planners wait too long, of course, they may find themselves without a significant role to play in an organization that has an effective marketing program.

Some barriers can be anticipated by a planning staff attempting to expand into marketing. Since the marketing function must be incorporated into overall management, where planning has not been, this will represent a significant shift in relationships. The threat that the planning staff may represent to others in making such a major upward climb may arouse some resentment. Planners should tread carefully in establishing new working relationships with other functions.

PLANNING, PUBLIC RELATIONS, AND DEVELOPMENT

The most complex situations for developing a marketing program will arise in organizations that have two or three of these three functions already in place. Where one already has been executing the marketing function in all but name, many difficulties of accommodation may have been overcome already. Where marketing is truly being introduced for the first time, however, there are likely to be significant conflicts and "border wars." However neatly each of the three functions has been defined and has related to the others in the past, marketing will put a severe strain on their interactions.

The choice as to which of the three should be given the responsibility for marketing, or whether new staff personnel should be brought in, is a matter of judgment for each organization. Ideally, the staff that has demonstrated the greatest interest and competence in dealing with behavior, causes, and impacts should be chosen. In theory, this should be the planning staff, though reality may differ in some institutions. Since planning would be the function most likely to be displaced by a marketing program, it should be considered first, if only to recognize that something will have to be done about it.

In some organizations, a committee approach may work. Rather than absorb any or all of the public relations, development, and planning functions into a new marketing department or staff, the three could join with administration in being the marketing function, with each contributing staff support as appropriate. However, remember such admonitions as:

"Too many cooks spoil the broth," or
"A camel is a horse designed by a committee."

But such an approach should be considered carefully before it is adopted.

However marketing is incorporated into the organization's governance and program, it will have to maintain effective working relationships with public relations and development, and even planning if it remains as an architectural function. A committee approach may be used rather than subordinating the three to marketing. On the other hand, it must be recognized that a marketing program cannot be optimally effective unless the three functions of planning, public relations, and development are carried out with a marketing perspective.

SUMMARY

Marketing must be absorbed by and incorporated into five components of the organization to be optimally effective. It is not a remote staff function but a philosophy and practical approach that must be accepted and supported by the governance of the institution, including owner, board, administration, medical staff, and political officials as appropriate. Similarly, it must be understood, accepted, and *practiced* by those who carry out the organization's function, who are its product. These include department managers, supervisors, and employees at all levels, although their involvement may be informal and/or representative.

The development function is specifically a marketing activity, though it may retain a separate identity if you wish. In some organizations, the development staff actually may take on the marketing function. In any case, specific roles and responsibilities for marketing and development must be delineated clearly and completely.

Public relations, like development, also is a marketing activity that can retain a separate identity if desired. In some organizations, P.R. staff members may well be qualified for and interested in the entire marketing function. They should take it on only if they are willing and capable of covering behavior as well as image, dealing with actions by the organization as well as its words, and with communications not only outward but inward. Again, specific roles and responsibilities relating and coordinating marketing and public relations are critical.

Planning figures to be absorbed completely into an effective marketing program unless it is restricted to architectural responsibilities. In theory, planners should be closest to the knowledge and skills required for marketing. In practice, whether they are competent and interested will have to be determined. For their own sakes, they'd be better off becoming so, rather than remaining aloof. In any case, all three functions are important to marketing and whether separate or absorbed will have to be coordinated effectively.

Chapter 12

Marketing Marketing

Because there is widespread misunderstanding of what marketing is all about, there is likely to be resistance ranging from some to substantial to its use by health care organizations. So, too, because marketing can be and has been used to misguide consumer choice and pander to "irrational" consumer behavior, there is likely to be some feeling that it is an unacceptable discipline for the health field. If you plan to use marketing, you may have to devote some initial attention to convincing various interests that it is acceptable and worth its costs.

In keeping with the principles of marketing, to "sell" a marketing program it is necessary first to identify the nature and attitudes of those you wish to "buy." Who are the organizations and individuals whose attitudes or behavior toward marketing should be predicted and/or influenced? What are their motivations for their current attitudes and probable behavior if you ignore them? What kind of product can you make of your marketing program to make it acceptable to those whose acceptance or support is critical? How can you communicate effectively to those whose attitudes and behavior make a difference?

MARKETS

The people and organizations you're likely to be concerned about include groups within and outside the organization. Among inside publics are likely to be one or more of the following:

- governing and/or advisory boards
- medical staff, referral physicians
- employees
- volunteers, auxiliaries

- managers of affected departments

Among outside groups are likely to be:

- customers—current and prospective patients
- planning and regulatory agencies
- rate-setting or reimbursement organizations
- accreditation and certification bodies
- donors

ATTITUDES/BEHAVIOR

Without your intervention, one or more of these groups may be able to damage, hinder, or reduce the effectiveness of your marketing efforts. Governing board members may reject the program or reduce your budget for it. Medical staff members may lobby against it, refuse to cooperate, or defect, to say nothing of causing you to lose your job. Employees may sabotage your efforts through resistance or halfhearted cooperation. Volunteers and auxiliaries may reduce their contributions. Managers of affected departments simply may fail to coordinate effectively or motivate their employees appropriately.

Customers may be turned off by some aspects of marketing and reduce their use of your services. Planning and regulatory agencies may disagree with your market objectives or strategies and refuse to approve certificate-of-need applications. Rate-setting and reimbursement organizations may refuse to pay for your marketing efforts. This particular threat usually can be averted simply by using another label: program planning or development instead of marketing; community or public relations or communications rather than advertising. Accreditation or certification bodies may withhold or threaten to withdraw their blessing (see Chapter 14). Donors may refuse to contribute to what they regard as unseemly activities.

PRODUCT

To avoid such untoward resistance and its consequences, you must be sure your marketing program truly does offer benefits worth the perceived costs to all those affected. Inside groups will require some communications that clarify to them the purposes of your marketing efforts. Their responses to your market audit should indicate their current attitudes toward marketing, if you ask them. By pointing out your intention to better identify the needs of the community and translate them into use, you should increase the acceptability of marketing within your organization.

Outside groups also will have to be informed better about what marketing in general and your program particularly are all about. By pointing out the virtues of market positioning in terms of optimum cost and quality to your markets, you should be able to reduce the potential opposition of planning, regulatory, and rate-reimbursement bodies. If donors have fixed ideas as to what you should do with their money (e.g., a new wing named after them), you may indeed lose some contributors if your market analysis suggests superior choices. You often will be better off without such donations, however, since you have to bear the long-run operational consequences of misdirected capital investment, even if the capital is donated.

ETHICAL ISSUES

There are basically three areas in which ethical issues arise with respect to marketing. First are questions as to the effects of marketing activities. Will they manipulate consumer demand to benefit the institutions with no concomitant benefits to the public? Will they simply exacerbate competition and raise cost of health care? The second area is advertising. Is it ethical for health care organizations to advertise? What can they communicate about themselves without breaking the bounds of decency? Third is research. Is it ethical to probe into human motivation?

IMPACTS

The questions of what health care organizations should market legitimately has been raised on occasion. Examples of surgery for convenience such as breast enlargement and psychosurgery are cited. Drug therapy designed to make healthy people feel better or happier is another potential issue. Abortions are a special case. Is it truly ethical for a health care organization to conduct amniocentesis on a pregnant woman to determine the sex of the fetus, followed by an abortion if it's the wrong one? Are there no circumstances under which it would be unethical for an organization to supply an abortion on demand?

It has been argued for some time that health care has too good a market already. People rely on it rather than first protecting their own health or caring for many minor conditions themselves. The public tends to believe that there's a medical solution for any problem. Pandering to such a belief could raise the utilization and costs of health care. Should hospitals attempt through marketing to lure away patients from a colleague already beset by low occupancy?

ADVERTISING

Most of the attention given to ethical issues in marketing has focused on advertising. This is due in part to the fact that most people equate the two. Another factor is the traditional resistance of the medical profession to advertising, its conviction that calling attention to oneself is unethical. However, the Federal Trade Commission in late 1979 ordered the American Medical Association to let its member physicians advertise fees and compete for patients. It did say the AMA could write its own prescription for advertising and could enforce reasonable ethical guidelines to prevent deceptive or unsubstantiated claims. The Supreme Court's earlier approval of lawyer advertising indicated the AMA's appeal would meet the same fate. Presumably, health organizations that compete with or depend on physicians are affected by the same ruling.

The American Hospital Association spent much time and effort examining this question. Its code of ethics on the subject was published in 1978. Basically, it called for:

- truthfulness/accuracy, no misleading information
- avoidance of self-aggrandizement
- no quality comparisons with others
- no claim of prominence, bestness, bigness
- no promotion of individual professionals

It recognized that advertising, bound by such strictures, was perfectly appropriate in such areas as:

- informing the public about services available, hours, etc.
- educating the public regarding health, including promoting your own health education efforts
- accounting to the community what you've done with its "trust," e.g., annual reports
- soliciting financial support for capital fund drives (but not political support in lobbying efforts)
- recruiting employees—perhaps even physicians for hospital-based positions

One specific example of an advertising problem has been the identification of physicians by specialty in the Yellow Pages telephone directories. While hardly a major "advertising" effort, this was resisted for years by physicians themselves because of their fear that such information would promote "shopping" behavior by patients. They felt individuals would tend to diagnose themselves and select a specialist accordingly, rather than see their family physician who could do a better job of diagnosis and then select a specialist for referral if necessary. Physicians also feared such shopping behavior would promote fragmentation of services and unnecessary use of specialty care.

Those fears have been largely borne out. Individuals do shop increasingly for their sources of care, picking their own specialist, though probably through word of mouth as often as through Yellow Pages advertising. Such shopping perhaps is an inevitable result of declining faith in medical practitioners and increased consumerism generally. How much advertising has contributed to the shopping phenomenon is not at all clear.

The fact that Health Maintenance Organizations do advertise heavily presents an interesting context for discussion of the ethics of advertising. HMOs engage in advertising out of necessity, and in the tradition of health insurance rather than health care delivery organizations. Yet what they are advertising and marketing to the public is, in most cases, an alternative source of care, not a new means of financing it. Much of the traditional opposition to HMOs or predecessor prepaid group practices by the medical profession has arisen from their practice of advertising. While such advertising calls attention to an organization rather than to an individual physician, this merely means the organization is claiming to deliver medical care, which physicians regard as another unethical practice.

While HMOs have obtained only a small share of the total market (3 to 4 percent), their effects are far beyond their numbers. In many areas, their market shares are 10, 20, or 30 percent, and alternative health care delivery organizations have felt their impact severely. Efforts to exempt HMOs from control under certificate-of-need or rate-regulation programs could give them substantial competitive advantages in the future, on top of the federal support and required employee choice laws that help them already.

The strongest justification for developing an active marketing program is the fact that a competitor has done so and is benefiting from it to your detriment. This, in effect, is what has happened among successful HMOs, which were not prevented from developing marketing and advertising programs by ethical or financial constraints. Where they have aggressively advertised and otherwise promoted their product, their competitors have been virtually forced to go along.

Few HMOs have entered into coordinative planning and development arrangements with their colleagues in the health field, so competition still is the order of the day. In fact, such competition is being promoted actively by federal health and trade policies. Whether this policy is consistent with the anticompetitive constraints of certificate of need and rate setting is open to question, but for a government that tries to get us to stop smoking while subsidizing tobacco growers, inconsistency is not foreign.

If HMOs are not governed by the same rules regarding competition, coordination, or the ethics of advertising, we must wonder how long the rest of the health care system can be constrained. It may well be that future advertising policies and practices of health organizations will approach the kinds of cartoons that have been used by some analysts to dramatize the issue:

- flashing neon signs indicating that patients can LIMP IN and LEAP OUT of physical rehabilitation programs
- weekend specials on appendectomies and tonsillectomies
- cut-rate specials on abortions advertised in the media
- placards describing the latest organ that can be transplanted here

RESEARCH

The ethical issues in market research are related first to the propriety of finding out things about people, and second of using what you find to take advantage of knowledge of human motivation to manipulate behavior. Ethical issues related to probing individuals' psyches are common to all industries, although health care organizations may be especially sensitive. The use you make of what you learn about human motivation may be geared to your advantage rather than to your market's but by definition you must offer your customers something they at least want.

Some particular ethical issues arise in regard to identification of the researcher. Whether you use an outside consultant, volunteers, students, or your own staff to carry out a market audit, for example, do you make clear to those outside the institution that you're asking questions in the interests of the organization? Do you risk biasing the answers if you identify yourself? In general, you never should mislead the public as to who you are, for both ethical and practical reasons. If respondents ask who's sponsoring the research, your surveyors should be instructed to identify your organization. If the question comes up as to why you're asking questions, you should give a truthful answer. Since the truth should be that you are hoping to make your organization more responsive to the needs and preferences of consumers, the answer should not damage your cause.

What you seek to learn from people should be understood in the same terms. The essence of marketing is, most simply, to discover what the market wishes to purchase and arrange to supply appropriate responses to those wishes. While understanding human motivation in some ways may enable you to take advantage of people (e.g., understanding the sex appeal of convertibles), behavior rarely is so irrational that you don't have to offer a legitimate benefit to win their trade (look what happened to convertibles!).

The use you make of what you learn is ultimately a matter of your choice. Markets can be misled by slanted advertising and glossy packages, where purchase decisions are optional and competitive choices fairly similar. As health care organizations increase the scope of their services toward holistic health, the possibility of misuse of marketing techniques probably increases. The more unsure the consequences of specific services, the more careful you have to be in describing their value to the public. The idea of a moneyback guarantee if customers aren't satisfied, already being used by one hospital in Ohio, is one way of "keeping you honest."

Where individuals have a voluntary choice of options, and aren't lied to through false or slanted advertising, marketing says they will buy only what gives them a worthwhile benefit in return. They may be mistaken in their expectation of benefits the first time, and occasionally as the result of advertising, but they are unlikely to make the same mistake twice. Health care organizations depend on long-term trust and loyal relations with their markets, and should avoid unethical practices for practical as well as moral reasons.

ADVANTAGES AND ARGUMENTS

Once you have designed your marketing program in response to your understanding of the groups whose support or acceptance you need, you can begin to design your promotional efforts. Like any marketing effort, however, the product (benefits to your organization and persons you're concerned about) and price (cost to the organization and them in time, money, lost power, etc.) must be developed or at least designed first. Promotional activities then should be geared to describing what you've designed as you see it from the perspective of the groups whose support you need.

One advantage you can cite for marketing is the comprehensive data base it offers through the market audit. While what you discover may not always please you or the specific publics you're concerned with, it should provide a useful information base for any of your planning and development, whether or not you use further marketing concepts and techniques. The understanding of causes, behavior, and impacts, together with your analysis of environment and competition, should point toward the advantages of other marketing analysis and strategies.

The advantages of a behavior rather than a need basis for maintaining, developing, or reducing programs ought to be clear to groups within and without your organization. Where you have found yourself in difficulty in the past because of gearing programs to what professionals were convinced was needed, the opportunities available through behavior-based development should represent a positive and significant contrast. The cases in Part IV illustrate some of the advantages of assorted marketing analysis and strategies, while also pointing out some disadvantages of being ignorant of them.

The strongest argument you probably can make for a marketing program is that you've always been engaged in one, though probably unconsciously or no more than implicitly. An explicit, overall marketing approach rather than incidental, fragmented efforts should have the appeal of all "organized" vs. "disorganized" efforts. Where the label "marketing" is unacceptable, it can be avoided easily. What marketing covers is simply good program planning and development, so this can be an optional label.

Another strong argument is the competitive reality that marketing, when employed well, does work to the advantage of those who use it. Actual or potential examples of effective marketing by you or by your competition should strengthen your persuasive efforts. The pride most organizations take in being at the forefront rather than the rear of developments in health care should aid you also. A simple count of the pieces of literature on the subject over the last few years should demonstrate the strength of current interest in marketing. (Count, for example, the number of health journal citations in my first book vs. this one.)

Where resistance to your arguments remains strong, you can employ group processes. Those who are least comfortable about the use of marketing by health care institutions might be the very persons who should be included or at least represented on your marketing committees and task force. Some hands-on experience with marketing in the analysis of some problem or development of a program should help you convince the reluctant of its nature and value. By involving them, you give them an opportunity to protect the interests, whether economic or moral, they feel are threatened.

MARKETING EVALUATION

The strongest argument you can make for the use of a comprehensive marketing program is a specific successful example of its effectiveness in your organization. This suggests that you might wish to employ an incremental approach to marketing your marketing program, much as was suggested for the market audit. The audit itself is a first increment, but you may try introducing further marketing efforts on a program-by-program or segment-by-segment basis. You can, in effect, conduct control vs. experimental group trials of marketing vs. nonmarketing on comparable programs or segments to test the effects of your efforts.

To some extent, an incremental approach may be necessary if you cannot obtain the personnel, information, and financial resources to institute a comprehensive program. By focusing your marketing efforts on specific problems, you can hone your own skills and whet the appetites of your critical publics for more. It is not necessary to choose your biggest market problem, threat, or opportunity to demonstrate with, however, unless you are convinced it is amenable to success. The biggest challenges are not necessarily the best starting points in any field of endeavor, hence the maxim: walk before you run. (See Chapter 8.)

Careful evaluation of your marketing results, through what by then will be a *marketing* audit, should identify both the desired and perhaps some undesired consequences of your marketing efforts. Marketing has costs, in time and resources, so it should produce demonstrable benefits. You should focus a certain amount of attention on determining not only what positive changes have occurred in your market relations but which specific marketing efforts produced or at least promoted such changes. You don't want to be found in the circumstances of a physician who tries dozens of therapies on a patient and finds that, although the patient recovers, no one knows for sure why. (See Chapter 16.)

As you increase your own skills and confidence in marketing, and its acceptance among your organization's publics, you may want to extend its concepts and techniques into other applications. While initial efforts may focus on market relations with patients and physicians, you may find that personnel and labor relations offer appropriate challenges as well. It might be particularly inappropriate to claim you are "marketing" to your own employees, but the basic notions are applicable. Wherever you have significant relations with individuals and organizations that can be understood, predicted, and influenced in terms of exchange transactions, there's the promise that marketing can help. The more you learn about it and use it, the more applications you'll probably find for it. The more successful your applications are, the greater acceptance it will generate.

SUMMARY

The marketing of a marketing program begins with identifying your markets: the individuals and organizations whose acceptance or support is important. These include internal groups (physicians, employees, boards, volunteers) as well as external (patients, regulatory and reimbursement agencies, accreditation bodies, and donors). Their current attitudes and behavior should be identified, problems or threats specified, and objectives targeted for change.

To develop a marketing strategy for your marketing program itself (product) you first must ensure that it promises significant benefits or few threats (price) to your publics. Ethical issues regarding marketing for health care organizations should be identified and addressed—specifically issues of marketing impacts, advertising, and research. The behavior of other health organizations, including HMOs, should be examined for cues as to what issues are involved in using vs. ignoring marketing.

The promotion you use for the program you develop should focus on the specific advantages that such a program offers the organization, the concerned interests, and the community at large. The specific values of marketing audit information, behavior rather than need-based planning and development, and making explicit and coordinated what you've been doing in an implicit, disjointed manner should be cited. The consequences of engaging in vs. ignoring marketing, especially where competitors use it, should be discussed.

The best argument for marketing is that it works. You may choose to show that it works in small ways, enhancing your skills as well as building arguments. A series of small successes may suffice. Effective evaluation via a marketing audit will demonstrate what works and what doesn't and, you hope, why. By involving concerned interests in designing and implementing your marketing program, you may not only enhance their acceptance, but also take advantage of their insights.

Readings

Ethics

Aden, G. "Hospitals Must Lead the Way in Meeting Public's Demands." *Hospitals, JAHA* 51:22, November 16, 1977.

Bezilla, R., et al. "Ethics in Marketing Research." *Business Horizons,* April 1976, p. 83.

Cunningham, R. "Of Snake Oil and Science." *Hospitals, JAHA,* April 16, 1978, p. 79.

Egdahl, R., and Walsh, D. (eds). *Health Services and Health Hazards: The Employee's Need to Know.* New York: Springer-Verlag, 1978.

"Health Care Advertising and Marketing: The Lady or the Tiger?" Ibid., Chapter 2, p. 38.

Giller, D. "Hospitals Face a Marketing Future," Chapter 11 in Egdahl and Walsh, op. cit., p. 312.

Lurie, R., and Bilbo, R. "HCHP Success and Failures in Communicating Information to Its Publics." Chapter 14 in Egdahl and Walsh, op. cit., p. 393.

Marshall, C. "Ethics Aspect of Advertising Debated." *Modern Healthcare,* April 1977, p. 48.

Miller, R. "Hospital Advertising Guidelines Require Immediate Consideration." *Hospital Management Communications* 2:13, 1978, p. 2.

Oliphant, C. "Making Advertising a Part of the Hospital's Communications Program." *Hospital Management Communications* 2:13, 1978, p. 4.

Peck, R. "Do Yellow Pages Make You See Red?"*Medical Economics,* August 22, 1977, p. 114.

Ralston, R. "Hospital Advertiser Denies Existence of Marketing Program." *Modern Healthcare,* October 1977, p. 70.

"Unique Ad Strategy Increases Use of Sunrise Hospital on Weekends." *FAH Review,* June 1977, p. 47.

Will, G. "Abortions as Commodity, Not Medicine." *The Washington Post,* 101, June 25, 1978, p. 7.

Wolinsky, H. "Hospitals Try Sell Tactics." *Today,* Special Report, June 12, 1977, p. 1.

HMO Advertising

Bilbo, R. *Marketing PrePaid Health Care Plans.* Washington D.C: U.S. Department of Health, Education, and Welfare, 1972.

Collins, J. "Maintaining an HMO by Marketing to Its Members." *Medical Group Management* 24:5, September/October 1977, p. 40.

Galiher, C. and Costa, M. "Consumer Acceptance of HMOs." *Public Health Reports* 90, March-April 1975, p. 106.

Gumbiner, R. *HMO, Putting It All Together,* St. Louis: Mosby, 1975.

Kress, J., and Linger, J. *HMO Handbook.* Rockville, Md.: Aspen Systems Corp., 1975.

Linde, K. and Strumpf, G., "Information Barriers to HMO Development." Chapter 15 in Egdahl and Walsh, op. cit., p. 416.

Marketing of Health Maintenance Organizations, Washington, D.C.: Bionetics Research Labs, Inc., 1972.

Miseneth, P. "Marketing Ambulatory Care." *Hospital Progress,* March 1978, p. 58.

Strehlow, J. "Marketing a Medical Group Practice." *Medical Group Management* 25:6, November-December 1978, p. 23.

Marketing Audit/Evaluation

Analyzing and Improving Marketing Performance. New York: American Management Association Report #32, 1959.

Bauer, R., and Fenn, D. "What Is a Corporate Social Audit?" *Harvard Business Review,* January/February 1973, p. 37.

Crisp, R. "Auditing the Functional Elements of a Marketing Operation." In AMA, op. cit., p. 16.

Felton, A. "Conditions of Marketing Leadership." *Harvard Business Review,* March-April 1956, p. 119.

Kelley, E.J. *Marketing Planning and Competitive Strategy.* Englewood Cliffs, N.J.: Prentice-Hall, Inc., 1972, p. 121, ff.

Kotler, P., and Lopata, R. "The Marketing Audit." In Britt, S. (ed.), *Marketing Manager's Handbook.* Chicago: Dartnell Corp., 1973, p. 1074.

Kotler, P. *Marketing Management.* Englewood Cliffs, N.J.: Prentice-Hall, Inc., 1967, pp. 596-602.

Oxenfeldt, A.R. *Executive Action in Marketing.* Belmont, Calif.: Wadsworth Publishing Co., 1966, p. 746 ff.

"The Marketing Audit as a Total Evaluation Program." AMA op. cit., p. 25.

Rothman, F. "Intensive Competitive Marketing." *Journal of Marketing,* July 1974, p. 10.

Sessions, R. "What a Soundly Conducted Marketing Audit Can Accomplish." AMA op. cit., p. 20.

Shuchman, A. "The Marketing Audit: Its Nature, Purposes and Problems." Ibid., p. 11.

Smith, C. "Standards for Appraisal of the Marketing Audit." Ibid., p. 48.

Tirmann, E. "Should Your Marketing Be Audited?" *European Business,* Autumn 1971, p. 49.

Cases in Market Analysis and Strategy

This section includes four cases describing market analysis and strategy employed by hospitals and four cases on innovative program development. The first four are examples of how the principles and techniques of marketing are or might be used by hospitals to increase the success of their current programs. The last four describe how the same principles and techniques are or might be used to diversify into new program areas.

The success of inpatient-oriented institutions is determined primarily by the ability to recruit and maintain an adequate referral base. Each physician or referral agency represents the probable source of large numbers of patients. While marketing to such sources is an essential factor in the success of inpatient programs, it is well-developed and most often effectively practiced already.

The opportunities for diversification—the new frontiers of program development—are almost entirely outpatient or even nonpatients. The significance of this fact lies in the extent to which individual consumers determine whether, how often, and where they will go for specific services. There is a referral network for many of these services, but it is likely to be an insufficient basis for cultivation of adequate utilization. Competition in the innovative service areas is likely to be fiercer, and physicians have less control over patients potentially interested in such services.

The types of offerings range from fairly close to traditional medical services to quite a ways away. Outpatient surgery, freestanding emergency medical services, and basic primary medical care programs are relatively mild innovations. They represent incremental shifts away from conventional hospital inpatient and outpatient services or private physician practice. As such, they have been the first to be developed, since the more familiar is likely to be tried first.

Many such programs have been developed successfully, and publicized as a result. Many more have been failures, and rarely heard from. Each has

brought with it the added dimension of having to attract at least some patients directly. None have been able to rely on existing referral networks for
an adequate supply of customers. As a result, where developers of such programs have done effective jobs of market analysis and strategic development,
either consciously or intuitively, they by and large have succeeded. Where
mistakes were made, usually by not using marketing techniques at all rather
than making erroneous judgment, failure has followed.

Beyond the development of conventional, ambulatory medical services
(Chapters 17, 18, and 19) there lie a vast number of partially medical and
nonmedical health services. An example of such a service is provided in
Chapter 20, but countless others are available. All have in common a greater
degree of consumer control over use of, and a reduced ability to rely on,
existing medical referral networks.

Generally speaking, the further a health organization strays from conventional medical services, the greater the competition and the greater the consumer control. Without the monopoly power of medical licensure, it is difficult for health organizations to claim an exclusive right to specific services.
For nonmedical health services, competitors may include not only other
health organizations but commercial and social service organizations as well.

Chapter 20 describes a hospital's developing a program that competes not
only with private physicians but also with commercial hearing aid dealers.
This hospital enjoyed substantial competitive advantages, but such superiority is likely to be rare in other opportunities for diversification.

The combination of demographic (aging of the population) and psychographic (greater interest in self-actualization and taking responsibility for
one's own health) create a host of diversification opportunities:

- day care and other semicustodial arrangements for the elderly
- periodic short stays for chronic disease and disabled patients
- educational/motivational programs in protecting one's own health, such
  as weight-loss clinics, giving up smoking, guided exercise
- mental health care, ranging from acute inpatient to halfway houses and
  outpatient counseling
- positive health programs, including education in self-care, self-awareness,
  positive wellness, etc.

The next few decades are likely to see the growth of regional health systems, linking medical care programs to each other and to other health-related
programs. Diversification, coordination, and horizontal and vertical integra-
tion already are well under way. All will entail, either consciously or not, the

use of marketing concepts. All will require identifying what others are interested in and what you can offer them in exchange for what interests you.

The cases here illustrate how this basic concept of exchange affects the development of new programs, either positively or negatively. In your reviewing of these examples of diversification opportunities, it should be clear that all will require establishing new patterns of behavior. Some involve new services not likely to be available now, but address needs that, if perceived, people must be coping with somehow. Others will require that individuals switch from one source of services to another. If your program is to succeed, you must offer something that will be viewed as superior to the competition by at least a significant segment of the market.

Diversification should not be pursued for its own sake, any more than should expansion. Development of new, innovative services will involve new risks as well as the potential for new rewards. Any such development should be pursued in the confident expectation that both the community and the organization will be significantly better off as a result. Each specific opportunity should be followed up when it offers the best chance for the greatest success.

Chapter 19 presents a generic model for approaching the development of any new noninpatient service, although it focuses on primary care. The principles that apply for any program dependent primarily on consumer choice are applicable universally. The techniques likely to be useful in researching, analyzing, and developing a primary care program will be equally applicable to any of the opportunities for diversification listed earlier.

Cases are never quite thorough or typical enough to provide complete insight or to offer a recipe for successful emulation in other circumstances. The examples here should help, however, in pointing out critical factors that should be considered and errors of omission or commission that should be avoided in order to enhance effective program development. It is in the best interests of each health organization and of the public at large that marketing be done well. It is hoped that these examples of both good and bad marketing will enable readers to learn from the experience of others.

The book closes with a chapter (Chapter 21) devoted to brief discussions of some of the major opportunities for new development in health services. All share a common trait: they require reexamining what business health care organizations are in, and assessing carefully the nature of the consumer market. Specific suggestions for how marketing techniques might be used in pursuing such new developments are included.

Chapter 13

Market Research Case

This case is based loosely on an analysis of market research efforts by a large multihospital corporation. The author acknowledges the contributions of his students: Keith Baldwin, Mike Boyd, and Natalie Novick in preparing an original case analysis, and that of Bill Tobin in supplying information and analysis on early drafts. The final version of this case has been augmented and altered by inclusion of experience of other market research efforts. It is meant to demonstrate a number of typical efforts and their strengths and weaknesses, rather than any specific approach.

Because market research provides the information base for marketing planning and programming, it is a critical first step. As described in Chapter 2, market research serves at both ends of the marketing program: identifying problems, threats, and opportunities, and evaluating results. This case includes the use of a specific research effort for both purposes.

THE REASON FOR THE PROJECT

Multihospital Corporation (MHC) operates a dozen hospitals in eight Western states. Each of these institutions is a large, full-service facility and operates independently, with modest guidance from the corporate headquarters and relatively minor sharing of services or coordination of activities with the other hospitals in the corporation. Having enjoyed modest but steady growth in occupancy, revenue, and outpatient visits for years, the corporation became concerned when all three categories seemed to level off during the 1970s.

A number of factors suggested the development of a corporate marketing program. The leveling-off of utilization and revenue figures suggested that previous plans based on expected continuing growth might have to be changed. Capital expansions carried out in anticipation of such growth now looked like overextension. The general feeling that the entire system was overbuilt suggested pressures on hospitals to reduce capacities unless they could expand the use of their existing capacity. Reimbursement based on presumptions of full utilization threatened financial disaster to hospitals that were underused.

While a number of executives in the corporation suggested immediate steps be taken, it was recognized that a full-scale marketing effort must begin, starting with an effective research program. Representatives of each of the hospitals were brought together to discuss what information should be sought. A consultant was employed to provide guidance on both the content and methodology of the research effort.

As a result of initial discussions, the research effort was divided into two major focuses, physicians and patients, categorized according to the major services offered by the hospitals: medical, surgical, obstetric, pediatric, and psychiatric inpatient care, plus emergency room and primary care clinic outpatient care. The initial research effort was aimed at discovering how individuals perceived the hospitals and their experience with them as well as what changes in the hospitals' overall programs and scope of services they would suggest.

A mail-return questionnaire was designed for distribution to patients and medical staff physicians. Each member of the medical staff was to get a questionnaire, while a sample of all patients discharged in September was considered adequate to test consumer opinions. Pretests of the questionnaire were carried out before the final format was chosen to be sure respondents could understand and would reply to questions.

THE INFORMATION SOUGHT

The patient questionnaire asked questions in seven categories:

1. demographic information: age, sex, race, residence of patient or respondent
2. referral chain: how patient happened to go to that particular hospital (e.g., family doctor, specialist, self-chosen, agency)
3. impressions of specific services and departments: admitting, nursing, room/service, lab, x-ray, food, business office, etc.
4. general impression: would they return to the same hospital, perceived overall quality, reputation of hospital in the community
5. knowledge and attitude regarding costs: familiarity with room charges, total bill, proportion covered by health insurance, perception of charges

6. suggestions for changes: what would they like to see different, what services should be added, which are unnecessary
7. major source of information on health: media, physician relatives, friends, agencies, etc.

Physicians were asked about their attitudes and behavior with regard to the hospital:

1. demographics: age, specialty, length of time on medical staff
2. other hospitals to which they refer patients, and an estimate of the number
3. perceived adequacy of staff, training, equipment, facilities, etc.
4. specific complaints
5. suggestions for changes in hospital's programs and services
6. general impression of the hospital as compared to other hospitals in the community (image)
7. major sources of information regarding health issues

The questionnaire was administered twice, in 1974 and 1978. This provided a basis for identifying problems (1974) and evaluating the success of steps taken to address those problems (1978). The combination of methods employed and the responses received does not always provide a clear picture, however.

PROBLEMS WITH RESPONSES

One significant problem was the rate of return. A total of 26 percent of all patients surveyed returned questionnaires in 1974, but only 18 percent in 1978. For physicians, the discrepancy was even greater: 44 percent returns in 1974 vs. 23 percent in 1978. This caused two problems. The low percentage of returns introduced substantial concern over potential bias. Could the respondents be considered truly representative of all patients and all physicians? Clearly some differences must exist if some persons responded and others didn't. Perhaps only those with strong feelings one way or another had sufficient interest to respond. Perhaps persons with complaints were more likely to fill out the questionnaire, or maybe less likely.

Normally, even though bias was a potential problem, the repetition of the survey at least should have detected trends. That is, if we can assume the bias was likely to be the same in 1978 as 1974, then any substantial change in the kinds of responses should be significant. A strong increase in positive or negative responses probably would reflect a true shift in the same direction for the entire population.

In this case, however, the drop in the percentage of persons responding cast doubt on even this assumption. Any change in the types of responses just as easily could be due to the dropout of responses of one type from 1974 to 1978. For example, it might be that of the 44 percent of physicians responding in 1974, half expressed positive comments and half negative. If, in 1978, the half who made positive comments simply lacked the motivation to fill out another questionnaire, while those with negative feelings still were motivated, the 23 percent response in 1978 easily could contain almost entirely negative responses. This would suggest a significant worsening of physician attitudes, while in reality there was no change.

A second problem arose in the analysis of results. In the initial runs, each factor in the questionnaire was treated independently. Thus, the results suggested the proportion of patients by religion, race, etc., the proportion who used services in different ways, the proportion who liked or disliked various aspects of the hospital's program, etc. However, no attempt was made to link results across factors; that is, no analysis was carried out to determine whether persons of one race or religion had different patterns of service use or different levels of satisfaction from others.

Similarly, MHC had no way of deciding whether physicians who were major admitters had different attitudes or suggestions from those of infrequent admitters. No distinctions between specialists and generalists or older vs. younger physicians were looked for, hence none were found. Fortunately, the data base was suited to such an internal analysis, and subsequent data runs detected some interesting distinctions.

Among patients, for example, walk-ins and those from the immediate neighborhood were more frequent outpatient visitors and slightly more frequent inpatients, but significantly less satisfied than their more distant counterparts. Older physicians tended to be generalists and have more admissions, but also held stronger views, both positive and negative, than their younger counterparts.

THE 'DON'T KNOW' FACTOR

Another problem arose with the proportion of respondents who failed to answer, or replied "don't know" to some questions. On one question, for example, the 1974 breakdown showed:

52 percent positive responses
25 percent negative
23 percent "don't know"

In 1978, this same question drew different responses:
64 percent positive
30 percent negative
 6 percent "don't know"

In interpreting these results, it was possible to conclude that the proportion of persons with positive attitudes went up significantly, from 52 percent to 64 percent—a positive result. However, it also was possible to concentrate on the increase in negative responses from 25 percent to 30 percent—a negative result. Neither was likely to be representative of actual change; the major difference was the decline in "don't knows," a result difficult to interpret. One way to avoid this equivocation is to inform respondents that their impressions, even if lightly felt, are important and that all questions should be answered. Another is to force answers by not providing "don't know" or other cop-out alternatives.

Some of the more interesting findings from the surveys included the indication that patients received most of their general health information from TV and radio rather than newspapers, but relied on friends and relatives for guidance on the choice of physician and hospital. This suggested that the general community image of the hospital and the experience patients had were likely to be more important public relations focuses than the advertising of specific services.

Physicians relied much more on newspapers and magazines and very little on radio or TV as sources of health information. Thus, image-building efforts aimed at physicians should concentrate on the written rather than spoken word.

One disappointing finding arose in one hospital area. In 1974, a significant number of patients in their responses expressed interest in an evening primary care clinic. When the hospital opened such a clinic in 1977, however, the response was very poor, and the clinic closed in 1978. A more careful analysis of the original returns suggested the reason for this inconsistency: most of the persons suggesting an evening primary care clinic in 1974 lived in the suburbs and were reacting to the lack of evening office hours among local physicians. However, these persons used the hospital only for inpatient care and didn't like to come downtown for care in the evenings; they really wanted an evening source of care in their own neighborhoods. Residents in the immediate area of the hospital continued to use the local emergency rooms because of better insurance coverage, or local free clinics because they were free.

The usefulness of the data in practice also suffered. For hospitals whose positive ratings apparently dropped, the results not only were embarrassing but also threatening. How does an administrator reply when asked: why did the proportion of respondents who rated your hospital "excellent" overall drop from 75 percent to 70 percent between 1974 and 1978? The administrators of hospitals whose 1974-78 "progress" appeared favorable tended to regard the results as a lucky break rather than truly significant. Similarly, those whose ratings dropped attached little significance to the decline. The fact that the corporation considered the results meaningful created a number of problems between headquarters and the individual hospitals.

ANALYSIS

As a market research effort, MHC's survey was a relatively sophisticated example compared to what most hospitals use. It employed a well-designed, easy-to-read questionnaire format and maintained that format for two surveys. This enabled the corporation to examine trends as well as get a one-time picture of how its hospitals were perceived by patients and physicians. By employing the same survey for all hospitals in the corporation, MHC built in a basis for comparison as well. The survey demonstrated that the corporation was truly interested in hospital patients and medical staff, so it presumably created some positive public relations effects.

Technically and practically, however, the surveys suffered from a number of drawbacks. No standards of acceptable quality were established for either survey, hence no uniform evaluation of returns was possible. Was a 90 percent good to excellent overall rating a positive or negative finding? While factual information was potentially useful (e.g., percent of individuals self-referred vs. those sent by physician), the quality ratings had no clearly accepted significance.

The biggest technical problem was the low and varying response rates. Patients submitted hundreds of returns, but they represented only 10 percent to 30 percent of potential respondents. Without even a small 100 percent sampling test, there existed no knowledge as to the opinions of nonrespondents. The possibility that changes from 1974 to 1978 represented shifts in self-selection of who replied rather than true changes in patient or physician attitudes toward the hospitals simply couldn't be dismissed. As a result, the responses failed to generate credibility among the hospitals and had little practical impact.

The greatest practical drawback was the fact that the survey was designed without any input from the hospitals themselves. As a result, administrators tended to discount the "ratings" they received and resented the corporations giving them so much emphasis. Few, if any, administrators believed the survey results and most felt threatened by the way the corporation used them.

Additional technical problems included the relatively small number of responses on some questions compared to the importance they were given. Few patients offered suggestions for changes, for example. If five persons out of 20 indicated a request for some service, this was reported as 25 percent of the sample, yet the five might represent only .5 percent of the 1,000 questionnaires distributed.

The technical and practical drawbacks complemented each other. Technical problems gave administrators an objective basis for disagreeing with the results and their meaning, although the true basis for their objection lay elsewhere. On the other hand, since the corporation was totally responsible for the survey, it had difficulty recognizing technical weaknesses and tended to be defensive about the results when dealing with administrators.

To improve future efforts, a number of changes were adopted. First, questionnaires were designed for the general population as well as for patients, for other physicians in the community as well as for medical staff members. This would enable the corporation to get a wider view of how its hospitals were perceived and estimate the feasibility of attracting new markets.

Second, the size of the samples was being reduced to 400 patients and 100 physicians per hospital. Serious efforts were to be made to obtain at least 90 percent return rates from these smaller samples. Combinations of mail, telephone, and personal visits would be used to assure high return rates. Hospital advisory board members and volunteers were to conduct interviews. This was expected to increase levels of community awareness in the institutions as well as save money on the surveys.

Samples were to be drawn on a systematic, stratified basis to be sure important segments of the market were represented adequately. Analysis was to concentrate on identifying differences in responses among specific segments as well as in overall ratings.

Representatives of each of the hospitals were included in designing the survey. Each was offered the opportunity to add questions unique to its own situation as well as using the standard questions. The comparison of one hospital to another was to be deemphasized in favor of each hospital's developing its own standards and program responses. The presumption voiced by the corporation was that all the hospitals were doing well, yet all could do better. The sense of the survey as a witch hunt had been reduced significantly.

CONCLUSION

Market research is a critical component of any marketing program. Done well, it can both smooth the acceptance of marketing as it is introduced and provide the basis for effective market analysis and strategy development. Done less than well, however, it can serve as a serious barrier to acceptance of marketing in general and provide unused results. It probably is better to start small, emphasizing technical quality and credibility, than to try to cover all purposes and issues in the first try.

It generally is best to agree upon the significance of responses before the survey is completed. This will tend to focus market research on subjects individuals are prepared to respond to, and prevent haggling over interpretation. On the other hand, some flexibility in interpretation of findings probably is necessary to achieving the acceptance and use of results.

The use of a consultant probably is a sound idea when entering into market research. However, the consultant should be used primarily to help design the survey technique and survey instrument. Content of the survey in terms of the questions to be answered and information to be provided should be decided by the health organization itself. Beware of canned surveys, however glossy, and focus on your own information needs rather than someone else's tried-and-true method for getting information somebody else wanted. Be sure you know how you will use the information you intend to get.

DISCUSSION QUESTIONS

1. Which markets are most interesting to you?
   - current patients?
     which services?
   - prospective patients?
     which services?
   - physicians—by type?
2. What behavior are you most interested in?
   - use of services (types, frequency)?
   - choice of source (reasons, satisfiers, and dissatisfiers)?
3. What knowledge are you most concerned about?
   - their awareness of health, symptoms?
   - their awareness of programs and services in the community?
   - their awareness of your programs and services?
4. Which attitudes most concern you?
   - their general attitudes regarding health?
   - their attitudes on the use of specific services?
   - their attitudes on specific sources of service?
5. Which knowledge, attitude, or behavior are you prepared to respond to or change?

Chapter 14
Market Audits:
Rural and Urban Examples

This chapter presents the contrasting situations of hospitals in rural and urban settings. Market audits were conducted in both locales, with expectably varying results. The juxtaposition of these dissimilar sets of circumstances provides an intriguing look at the small and the large and how they cope with their problems.

A RURAL AREA

Logan is the county seat of Marshall County, 150 miles from Capital City in its own state and 200 miles from a major metropolis in the neighboring state. There are some fairly large towns closer to Logan, one 30 miles to the northwest and another 60 miles to the south. Logan lies close to the interstate highway linking Capital City to the metropolis in the neighboring state.

Logan has a population of 11,000, the county as a whole about 20,000. The county population has been stable for the last ten years and projections suggest only modest growth to approximately 21,000 by 1985. Logan is projected to grow to only 12,500 by 1985. The city supports traditional retail and service businesses, as well as a lumber mill, paper mill, and apple processing plant.

The population of the area is predominantly white, with roughly 5 percent Hispanic and 4 percent native American minorities. The proportion of aged (over 65) is 12 percent, projected to increase to 15 percent by 1985. Roughly 25 percent of the population is under 15, but that proportion is projected to decline to 22 percent by 1985. Approximately 20 percent of the population is female, aged 15-44, with an equal proportion of males, leaving 23 percent aged 45-64 (see Table 14-1).

Logan Community Hospital (LCH) is the only hospital in the county, operating 50 acute care and 30 long-term care beds. It maintains an average

Table 14-1 Marshall County Population

	1977 (estimated)	1985 (projected)
under 15	5,000	4,620
15-44	8,000	8,400
45-64	4,600	4,830
65+	2,400	3,150
Total	20,000	21,000

occupancy of 64 percent in acute care beds and 80 percent in long-term care. Peak census levels usually occur in February or March and often fill virtually all available acute care beds. The long-term care beds generally are filled somewhat more in winter, and some local residents have sought nursing home care elsewhere because of the lack of empty beds.

The regional planning agency has set goals of 75 percent occupancy in rural hospitals and 85 percent in urban so as to achieve a statewide occupancy of 80 percent. It is pushing for consolidation of pediatric and obstetric units to achieve national guidelines of 20 beds for pediatrics, and 1,500 deliveries per year for obstetrics. Logan Community Hospital operates six pediatric beds, which have an average daily census of two. Its six obstetric beds also average a census of two, and handle about 240 deliveries per year. Both pediatric and obstetric beds are filled a number of times each year.

The residents of the county use hospital care at the rate of 160 admissions per thousand, and have an average length of stay of 5.0 days. They use 16,000 patient days of care per year, of which 70 percent (11,200) occur in LCH. In addition to its use by local residents, approximately 4 percent of LCH total patient days are used by out-of-county residents, primarily from Franklin County, just across the river (see Figure 14-1). The 30 percent of county use that goes to hospitals other than LCH includes 5 percent to Capital City, 5 percent to the neighboring state, 15 percent to Franklin County Hospital, and 5 percent to Eagle County Hospital.

Health indicators for Marshall County suggest that residents are about as healthy as the national and state average (see Table 14-2). Infant mortality rates have varied from 15 to 25 per thousand live births in the last five years, averaging 18.8. Last year the rate was 25. Overall mortality has been close to 9.0. Major causes of death are heart disease (showing a slight recent decline), cancer (increasing slightly), and cerebrovascular disease (also increasing). Accidental deaths are the fourth leading cause, the only specific one that has been consistently higher than state and national average over the last five years.

Figure 14-1 Area from Which Logan Hospital Draws

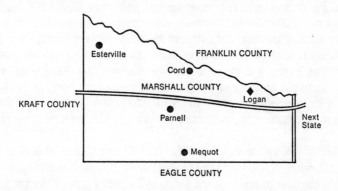

The Marshall County fertility rate has averaged 70 per thousand women aged 15-45 for five years but has been declining. Pediatric admission rates have averaged 60 per thousand, with an average length of stay of three days. Approximately 85 percent of resident obstetrical and 80 percent of resident pediatric admissions go to LCH. There were 1,856 medical/surgical admissions to LCH last year, with average length of stay of 5.5 days.

Of the 30 long-term care beds at LCH, 10 are designated as skilled nursing facility (SNF), with an average census of six, while the 20 intermediate care facility (ICF) beds have an average census of 18. The average stay in the SNF beds is 40 days and 320 days (for last year's discharges) in the ICF beds. No data exist on the proportion of Marshall County residents who use the LCH beds vs. long-term care facilities elsewhere.

Table 14-2 Mortality Rates Last Year

Cause of Death	Rate per 100,000 population		
	Marshall	State	U.S.
Heart disease	320	330	340
Neoplasms	195	170	180
Cerebrovascular	140	100	100
Accidents	70	50	50
Cirrhosis	20	15	15
Influenza/pneumonia	40	15	15
Suicide	10	13	12
Homicide	18	12	10
Arteriosclerosis	28	10	10
Other arterial	8	10	10
Infant mortality	25	15	16

Financial Data

Total inpatient acute care revenue last year was $2,044,000 against total expenses of $2,008,000 ($175 revenue per patient day vs. $172 expenses). If plans to gear allowable reimbursement to 75 percent occupancy had been implemented, revenue would have amounted to only $160 per patient day. The state rate-setting commission has been discussing calculating reimbursement rates based on occupancy standards, but hasn't implemented the idea. The hospital's emergency room handled 10,000 visits last year, up from 9,000 five years ago. Its average revenue per visit was $28; its average cost per visit $30.

Twelve physicians practice in Marshall County, nine of whom maintain offices in Logan. Five are general practitioners. Two are internists and two are surgeons, the four practicing as a group in Logan. Three of the general practitioners share the obstetric work. Of LCH's medical staff of 15, including three physicians from Franklin, none are under 35, seven are under 50, and four are at least 60. Only the three Franklin physicians have significantly reduced (about 40 percent) their admissions to LCH, but this reflects primarily a decline in their overall activity level rather than a decreased share for LCH. (See Table 14-3.)

Table 14-3 Market Share Analysis/Physician

	Age	Admissions to LCH	Town of practice*	Admissions to other hospitals (Estimated)	Percent to LCH
General practice	67	100	F	100	50
	62	150	P	50	75
	60	340	L	18	95
	55	280	L	15	95
	54	140	M	140	50
	52	100	F	150	40
	50	40	F	160	20
Family practice	45	120	L	80	60
	42	80	C	120	40
	40	60	E	140	30
	38	40	L	160	20
Surgeon	62	460	L	–0–	100
	40	180	L	20	90
Internist	38	140	L	60	70
	41	100	L	100	50

* C=Cord, E=Esterville, F=Franklin, L=Logan, M=Mequot, P=Parnell.

Table 14-4 Census Variation Last Year

	ADC	Peak	Low	Weekday	Weekend
Medical/surgical	28	45	10	30	23
Obstetrics	2	8	0	2	2
Pediatrics	2	9	0	2.2	1.5
	32	50	12	34.2	26.5
Skilled Nursing Facility	6	10	2	6	6
Intermediate Care Facility	18	20	16	18	18
	24	30	19	24	24

Table 14-5 Emergency Room Utilization Last Year

Visits per day		Visits per shift	
Sunday	36		
Monday	20	7-3	5
Tuesday	24	3-11	20
Wednesday	30	11-7	2
Thursday	26		
Friday	24		
Saturday	32		

Competition

For acute care, the only significant nearby competitor is Franklin County Hospital (FCH), an 80-bed facility 30 miles to the northwest, which provides a virtually identical set of services. It has two obstetricians and a pediatrician plus two surgical specialists on staff, although it operates no long-term care beds. Most of the cases from the Logan area that go to Franklin are for specialized obstetric, pediatric, gynecological, and other surgical care. FCH also operates its own primary care program, contracting with three family practitioners to provide on-site ambulatory care.

There is one nursing home in the area, offering 30 ICF and 60 custodial care beds. This home charges $3 less per day for ICF care than LCH and enjoys 95 percent average occupancy.

The regional Health Systems Agency has been enforcing a moratorium on the construction of acute care beds, citing the 64 percent occupancy at LCH and 60 percent at FCH as clear proof of a bed surplus. It has not adopted as an objective the closing of beds, although it has yet to perform its first Appropriateness Review, having achieved full designation only recently. Its efforts have been aimed more at direct cost containment through reimbursement limits in cooperation with the rate-setting commission.

Attitudes

Logan Community Hospital routinely monitors patient satisfaction by means of questionnaires mailed soon after discharge. By and large, returns indicate patients and their families are happy with the care they receive. Complaints primarily cite noise at night, unappetizing food, high costs, and air-conditioning problems. Special praise has been given the open visitor policy and pleasant surroundings. Feedback on the emergency room suggests some individuals are dissatisfied at not finding a physician available, long waits for lab and x-ray results, and high charges. Results of surveys of the long-term care patients indicate that the SNF patients essentially are happy, although some complain of the high charges, while ICF patients occasionally complain of the depressing hospital atmosphere.

A survey was conducted of Franklin and Marshall county physicians to determine where they refer their patients and why. The interviews indicate that the physicians on LCH staff send most of their patients to LCH, with only an occasional referral to the two major medical centers. Some indicated they sent surgical patients to Franklin on occasion when they felt the services of a specialist were called for. Two of the family practitioners indicated they referred all of their surgery away from Logan because they had problems with the two surgeons on the staff. They were reluctant to discuss the nature of the problems. They estimated the number of patients they sent to Franklin at 40 to 50 per year, but didn't know for sure.

Table 14-6 Market Share Analysis—Marshall County

Service	LCH%	FCH%	Other%
Medicine	90	2	8
Surgery	40	40	20
Pediatrics	80	8	12
Ob-Gyn	85	5	10
Average	71	14	12

Table 14-7 Financial Analysis

Service	Cost/day	Revenue/day	Free care & bad debts (%)
Medicine	145	130	15
Surgery	225	250	5
Pediatrics	165	160	5
Ob-gyn	165	150	10
Average	175	177	9

Table 14-8 Market Analysis

	% of LCH	% to LCH
Logan	66	80
Cord	8	60
Esterville	4	30
Parnell	10	70
Mequot	8	60
Out-of-area	4	
Total	100	

Follow-Up

In pursuing the results of its initial market audit, Logan Community Hospital followed up a number of leads. Analysis showed health status indicators varied no more than random variability would explain in most cases. Adjusting for age left most indicators equal to or better than U.S. averages. The high infant mortality rate was attributed to the tendency for small numbers to vary widely, not to a true decrease in health or the efficacy of natal care. Only the consistently higher than average mortality and morbidity due to accidental injuries was considered a significant indication of a problem. Logan was not sure that it was "its" problem in the sense of reflecting difficulties in its emergency service, however. The higher risk occupations and greater travel distance accounted for more of the discrepancy. This was reinforced by the higher than average proportion of heart attack victims who arrived dead at the hospital before any care could be given.

Organizational impacts of particular concern were the low return to reserve (net revenues) generated by operations and low occupancy, especially in obstetrics and pediatrics (33 percent). The prospect of occupancy-based reimbursement might force the hospital to close eight acute care beds. On the other hand, if it eliminated either pediatrics or obstetrics, it might lose much related utilization and incur the wrath of both medical staff and community. The slow population growth and future pressures on reducing inpatient utilization made it unlikely that occupancy would increase much by itself.

Behaviors of significant concern included the declining fertility rate that affected both obstetric and pediatric occupancy. While many persons using the hospital's emergency room were not emergency cases, both the community health and organizational impacts of this behavior were considered acceptable. Without the nonemergency volume, it would be harder still to finance the emergency room, and without it as a source of care, local physicians would be overtaxed in their offices. The medical staff and community felt the emergency room was an essential program, despite its problems.

Clearly, some of the physicians were not referring all the admissions they could to Logan. Market shares indicated more surgery admissions were going to Franklin than should, compared to all other services. While Franklin had a few more specialist surgeons, most of the referrals there could have been handled appropriately at Logan. With surgery the major net revenue producer, losses of surgical admissions were critical. Based on analysis of the medical staff, it would appear that the younger family practitioners and internists in Logan were underreferring. Moreover, the older surgeon probably was too busy and should add a partner to guarantee continuity as well as lighten his workload.

A number of causes for the behaviors of concern were investigated. Fertility rates had declined because of a number of social and economic developments, and no intervention by the hospital seemed reasonable. On the other hand, there were signs that fertility rates were starting upward again, and a significant increase in births could result, despite the anticipated decrease in women of child-bearing age.

Problems of low referrals appeared to be of two types, both related to personality rather than professional difficulties. The family practitioners and internists didn't like the busy surgeon or what they regarded as his out-of-date practices. They didn't get any referrals from the older physicians in town and didn't feel they had a loyal commitment to Logan. Recognizing that a number of these younger physicians were not terribly busy, the hospital considered contracting with them for emergency room coverage. This would aid the staffing problems there plus provide some automatic interactions between the older and younger physicians.

The second half of the physician situation was a threat rather than a problem. The busiest physicians and most active admitters were in their 60s and couldn't be expected to remain that busy forever. While a fair number of younger physicians had moved to the area, they didn't have the strong ties to Logan the older doctors did. Moreover, they tended not to admit as many of their patients or keep them there as long. From this purely practical viewpoint, Logan would like to add many more older loyal and frequently admitting physicians to its staff. In any case, some replacements for retiring physicians should be part of future strategies.

An opportunity might exist if more referrals from Franklin could be attracted. The lack of specialists and equipment at Logan kept such referrals at a minimum and contributed to outflow. The traditional dominance of general practitioners vs. specialists at Logan hindered recruitment. On the other hand, the older general practitioners were approaching retirement, and the family practitioners/internists were much more receptive to specialist recruitment. In the long run, Logan might be able to take advantage of this situation. Improving the emergency room operation (e.g., by using contract physicians rather than rotating coverage) could assist this effort.

Much of the ill feeling between generalists and specialists was caused by differences of opinion over credentialing or privileges. Generalists who had performed simple surgery and cared for some complex cases did not enjoy being told by specialists that they were incompetent to continue. Specialists did not feel comfortable having physicians who lacked their specialized training providing sophisticated services. Franklin was dominated by specialists who were seen as competitors for patients by the generalists at Logan.

Whether such a situation would be exacerbated or diminished through more formal working ties between Logan and Franklin was the subject of a fair amount of consideration by administrators of both hospitals. A few members of both boards, including three who served on both, suggested that informal discussions of the subject be begun. Before replacement of the older members of the two facilities became necessary, the advantages of joint, coordinated vs. separate, competitive operation should be investigated.

The growth in numbers of aged in the area was both an opportunity and a problem. It was an opportunity particularly for Logan since it had a long-term care facility in operation. Plans were under way to expand the number of beds, perhaps by converting unused acute care beds. Final plans were to be developed after discussion with Franklin and the regional health planning agency. The growth in aged also was a problem in that it would make Logan more dependent on government sources of income, Medicare and Medicaid, that had the tightest cost-based reimbursement and were going to move toward occupancy-based cost limits shortly.

The bad debt level was ascribed to both patients' lack of adequate health insurance coverage and low state funding for its medical coverage of indigents not eligible for Medicaid. There was no sign that the state planned, or was even willing, to increase its appropriations for this purpose, however. Sentiment was more toward controlling the state budget to increase no more than the Consumer Price Index. As long as hospital costs increased faster than the CPI, state support for hospital costs was likely to decrease, not improve.

DISCUSSION QUESTIONS

1. How would you describe the impact, behavior and cause results of the market audit performed by Logan in terms of problems, threats, and opportunities?
2. What problems, threats, and opportunities did Logan not perceive or misinterpret?
3. What additional information would have been useful to include in its audit?
4. If you were Logan, what market objectives would you establish in the short run? What goals in the long run?
5. What strategies could you employ to accomplish these objectives:
   - whose behavior
   - would change to what
   - for what reasons
   - with what impact

A MULTIHOSPITAL URBAN AREA

The following case describes a modified version of a real metropolitan area, served by six hospitals. The case focuses on a single institution in this multi-hospital community, starting with its audit and following through its discussion of objectives, adoption and implementation of strategies, and evaluation of results. Since it is a specific, real situation, there is a limit to how many general principles can be illustrated or drawn from the one hospital's experience. The types of problems confronted and strategic choices open, however, tend to be typical. It is expected that readers will be able to find insights in addition to those suggested by the author.

Ocean City metropolitan area lies on both sides of Finger Lake, between the mountains and the sea. Its major transportation arteries are Interstate 110 running north and south, 410 running across the top of Finger Lake and along its eastern shore, and 610, which cuts across the lake, linking the eastern suburbs to Ocean City proper. The area prospers, based on an economy of boatbuilding, computer manufacturing, and agriculture, mostly fruit orchards.

Ocean City itself has grown about as large as its available space will permit, and future growth is projected primarily for the north and south suburbs, with eastside growth limited by the mountains. The fastest growing area actually is around Morgan City, whose 24,000 population is expected to double in 20 years as a nuclear power plant and research center, supporting an aluminum industry, continues to grow.

The Eastlake area is a suburban bedroom community of 60,000, with future growth limited by the mountains to the east. The unincorporated area of Southlake is expected to grow at a rate of 5 to 6 percent a year for the next five years, though long-range growth also is limited by the available land.

The health status of the area's population generally is sound, although some discrepancies exist between the affluent white populations in the suburbs and the poorer minorities in the core city. Use of health services is a little higher than national averages for physician visits, but significantly lower for hospital patient days (900 vs. 1,250 patient days per thousand). Both these realities are influenced by the Ocean City Prepaid Health Plan, an HMO to which 16 percent of the area population belongs.

Figure 14-2 The Six-Hospital Metropolitan Area

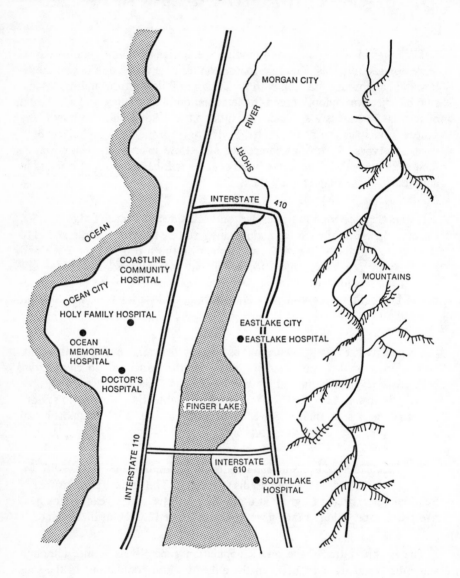

Table 14-9 Current Population Breakdown

Age	Male	Female	
0-14	36,858	35,631	72,489
15-44	56,413	58,422	114,835
45-64	25,116	30,362	55,478
65+	5,827	9,974	15,501
Totals	124,214	134,389	258,303

Current health care use rates include the following:

- hospital admissions rate: 150 per 1000 people

- average length of stay: 6.6 days

- obstetric admission rate: 1.1 per live birth

- fertility rate: 70 per 1,000 women 15-44

- physician visit rate: 4 per person per year

- emergency room visit rate: 300 per 1,000 per year

Patient origin data reflect the major markets and market shares for the area hospitals.

Table 14-10 Origin of Patients (Admissions)

Hospital	City	Suburbs	Morgan City	Elsewhere	Total
Coastline	2,610	1,240	2,400	50	6,300
Holy Family	12,270	950	500	1,000	14,720
Ocean Memorial	5,230	120	100	40	5,490
Doctors	5,210	160	200	110	5,680
Eastlake	520	4,120	400	0	5,040
Southlake	260	2,410	0	0	2,670
Totals	26,100	9,000	3,600	1,200	39,900

Table 14-11 Major Market Breakdown by Percent

Hospital	City	Suburbs	Morgan City	Elsewhere	Total
Coastline	41.4	19.7	38.1	0.8	100
Holy Family	83.4	6.4	3.4	6.8	100
Ocean Memorial	95.3	2.2	1.8	0.7	100
Doctors	91.7	2.8	3.6	2.0	100
Eastlake	10.3	81.7	7.9	0.0	100
Southlake	9.7	90.3	0.0	0.0	100

Table 14-12 Market Shares by Hospital, by Percent

Hospital	City	Suburbs	Morgan City	Elsewhere
Coastline	10.0	13.8	66.7	4.2
Holy Family	47.0	10.6	13.9	83.3
Ocean Memorial	20.0	1.3	2.8	3.3
Doctors	20.0	1.8	5.6	9.2
Eastlake	2.0	45.8	11.1	0.0
Southlake	1.0	26.8	0.0	0.0
Totals	100.0	100.1	100.1	100.0

Table 14-13 Current Utilization Data by Hospital

Hospital	Beds	ADC	Occupancy
Coastline	150	103.6	69.0
Holy Family	300	241.3	80.4
Ocean Memorial	180	105.3	58.5
Doctors	100	77.8	77.8
Eastlake	90	69.0	76.7
Southlake	100	58.5	58.5
Overall	920	655.8	71.3

Simultaneous examination of market shares and major markets indicate that Holy Family, with its 300 beds, serves as the major referral specialty care center for the area. Coastline enjoys a blend of major markets combining the city proper, suburbs, and Morgan City to the north. It receives the lion's share of admissions from Morgan, but relatively small shares of other markets. Doctors and Ocean Memorial are chiefly city-oriented, while Eastlake and Southlake are almost entirely dependent on the suburbs.

Of the six hospitals, only Holy Family offers acute psychiatric inpatient care, in a 20-bed unit. Only Southlake and Doctors do not offer obstetrics and pediatrics. The hospitals that have obstetric and pediatric services have suffered from recent declines in fertility rates.

While the local planning agency has been pressing for consolidation of obstetrics and pediatrics units in the area, none of the hospitals has volunteered to give up either of these services. Eastlake doesn't conform to National Health Planning Guidelines in that it has fewer than 20 pediatric beds in its unit. Of the four hospitals offering obstetrics, only Holy Family annually accommodates more than 1,500 deliveries, though the three other hospitals combined handle the same total.

Total hospital use in the area has changed only slightly in the past five years. Declines in obstetrics utilization are ascribed primarily to a dropping fertility rate, though some mothers have opted for home delivery. According to vital statistics reports, 3.4 percent of all births occurred outside the hospital last year, compared to 1.2 percent five years ago. The pediatric census drop also is an indirect result of fertility declines, although, increasingly, pediatric surgery is being done on an in-and-out basis. Had the number of ambulatory surgeries been included, an additional 1,304 partial patient days of care would have been recorded.

Table 14-14 Declines in Obstetrics and Pediatrics

Hospital	Ped Beds	ADC	Occ.	OB Beds	ADC	Occ.
Coastline	25	12.7	50.8	20	8.2	41.0
Holy Family	50	30.4	60.8	40	20.1	50.2
Ocean Memorial	30	10.8	36.0	20	7.8	39.0
Eastlake	12	5.7	47.5	10	3.1	31.0
Totals	117	59.6	50.9	90	39.2	43.6

Table 14-15 Patient Days in Hospitals

	-4	-3	-2	-1	last year
Total Pt. Days	231,412	233,647	241,233	236,710	239,367
Med-Surg	187,069	192,349	202,233	199,843	203,305
OB	15,631	14,877	14,616	13,912	14,308
Ped	28,712	26,421	24,384	22,955	21,754

Table 14-16 Impact of Changing Age Rates

Age	Current pt. days/1,000	Future population	Projected patient days
0-14	241	68,750	16,569
15-44	746	130,136	97,081
45-64	1,337	60,744	81,215
65+	3,547	25,179	89,310
Totals	5,871	284,809	284,175

The population is projected to shift significantly toward the older age range in the future. The potential impact is indicated by projections based on age-specific hospital use rates (Table 14-16). With this amount of utilization, the overall hospital census in the area would be 284,175 ÷ 365 = 778.6. If the current supply of beds remained at 920, overall occupancy would be 778.6 ÷ 920 = 84.6 percent.

Based on public reports submitted to the local voluntary rate review commission, the financial status of local hospitals would appear to be roughly as follows:

Coastline:	in the black two of last five years
Holy Family:	very strong
Ocean Memorial:	annual deficit running high
Doctors:	very profitable
Eastlake:	improving into black
Southlake:	deficits last three years

The other major factor in the health industry locally is the Ocean City Prepaid Health Plan, which has enrolled 16 percent of the local population. The use rate for the HMO population is a little over 475 inpatient days per thousand persons. While Ocean City Prepaid doesn't have a hospital of its own, most of its medical staff serves on the staff at Holy Family, and 87.4 percent of all the HMO's admissions go there.

Plans by the HMO call for growth to 25 percent of the market within ten years, and purchase or construction of its own hospital. This latter intention appears to be supported by the local planning agency even though the area as a whole is considered overbedded. The HMO tends to appeal most strongly to the younger married couples in the area (see Table 14-17).

Of the six local hospitals, Eastlake and Southlake are the newest, at six and ten years old respectively. Holy Family added one wing only four years ago but the balance of the facility is 22 years old. The Coastline and Doctors buildings are 15 while Ocean Memorial is 33. According to a recent Hill-Burton survey, the Ocean City facility is nonconforming and its accreditation by the Joint Committee on Hospital Accreditation is temporary. All other facilities are conforming and accredited.

Physician supply in the area generally has been healthy, with virtually all specialties represented. Primary care physicians are somewhat scarce on the east side of the lake, and particularly so in Morgan City, where only six are available for the 24,000 population. The seven psychiatrists in the area represent less than the national ratio, while both obstetricians and pediatricians theoretically are in oversupply. The only specialty not represented is that of physical medicine and rehabilitation; no rehabilitation program is offered locally.

Aside from Morgan City, the only other portions of the area not well-served are the core city area of Ocean City with a ratio of one physician per 6,000 persons and Southlake with one per 5,000.

Coastline Community Hospital

Focusing specifically on Coastline Community, it is a nonprofit community hospital built by a combination of Hill-Burton and community-raised funds 12 years ago. The 30-member board of trustees includes a number of local business executives, professionals, and social leaders, including three physicians from the medical staff.

The medical staff is relatively young, although the loyal core of key admitters all are over 50. While most of the staff members are board eligible or

---

Table 14-17 HMO Membership Age Breakdown

Age	Numbers	Percentage
0-14	11,820	28.6
15-44	20,044	48.5
45-64	7,728	18.7
65+	174	4.2
Totals	41,328	100.0

Table 14-18 Utilization of Coastline Units

Service	Beds	Admissions	LOS	ADC	Occupancy
Med-Surg	105	4,575	6.6	82.7	78.8
(ICU/CCU)	(6)	(249)	(4.1)	(2.8)	(46.7)
OB	20	881	3.4	8.2	41.0
Peds	25	844	5.5	12.7	50.8
Totals	150	6,300	6.0	103.6	69.1

certified, general and family practitioners are permitted limited surgical privileges. Most of the staff members have privileges at one or more of the other hospitals in town, chiefly at Holy Family.

Utilization of units at Coastline is barely adequate financially, and well below national standards (Table 14-18). Financially, daily adjusted revenue for inpatient care comes out at $4.62 above expenditures. Outpatient care, however, with a bad debt ratio of 16.3 percent, loses an average of $3.16 per visit. As outpatient volume increases, the losses generated in this area also have increased. The rate review commission governs only inpatient charges, but has been putting pressure on all local hospitals to keep their rates of increase below 10 percent a year.

Market Audit Analysis

From Coastline Hospital's perspective, some aspects of the market situation looked good, others not so good. It identified as problems its low occupancy, especially in pediatrics and obstetrics, and its losses from outpatient programs. The two major threats came from the growth of the HMO and the possibility that Morgan City might insist on developing its own hospital as its population continued to grow. Opportunities apparently available include: developing a physical rehabilitation program, waiting until population growth improves all local hospital occupancy, developing a competing HMO, and merging with Holy Family.

Each of these problems, threats, and opportunities was subjected to a behavior analysis; that is, Coastline attempted to identify whose behavior might be affected how if it made a specific change, or on whose behavior the success of a change depended. This initial focus on behavior of its markets would provide the basis for marketing strategy development and help it decide on the desirability or feasibility of alternative changes.

Problems

The apparent choices regarding low occupancy in pediatrics and obstetrics were to try to beef up the census, reduce beds, or close the units. The financial implications of each of these choices were examined. In general, increasing the census would have the best results, adding revenue and increasing efficiency. Closing the units would be next, since the losses incurred through operating these units were greater than the fixed costs of maintaining them unused. Reducing the number of beds would have no significant impact on costs since fixed costs would remain, but might result in some loss of revenue if there arose some occasions when all available beds were filled. If the obstetric and pediatric beds could be converted to medical/surgical use, some reduction in costs would be likely, but conversion costs would be high and occupancy levels in the existing M/S beds did not indicate a need for more beds.

The feasibility and desirability of the first two choices clearly were dependent on behavioral factors. Would obstetric/pediatric utilization generally increase so as to raise census to more efficient levels? Population and fertility projections suggested the opposite, and the growth of birth centers and home births cast further doubts on the prospects for increasing obstetric use. Could the hospital attract significant numbers of new admissions by competing with other hospitals? Here, too, prospects were not good. Medical staff loyalty in the area's hospitals was well-developed and no new pediatricians or obstetricians were expected to move to the area. Moreover, the other hospitals in the area also were seeking more pediatric and obstetric patients avidly.

The success of a decision to close either or both units also was subject to behavioral determination. How would the medical staff and current patients respond to such a closure? Some loss of gynecological surgery could be expected if obstetricians left. A survey of the medical staff indicated that most ob/gyn physicians specialized in either obstetrics or gynecology, so the expected loss of surgery was not estimated to be very high. However, a number of the hospital's surgeons indicated that they did a fair amount of surgery on children (e.g., ear/nose/throat) and would not take kindly to having to place their patients in two different hospitals. Pediatricians objected to losing obstetrics, as that would reduce the referrals of newborns to them in the hospital.

The biggest barrier to closing of obstetrics and/or pediatrics, however, arose out of Morgan City patients. The residents of that town used Coastline as their primary source of routine inpatient care, including much pediatrics and obstetrics. If Coastline closed either or both of these services, the citizens of Morgan City would increase their demand for a hospital of their own, citing the increased distance they would have to travel to the nearest source of that care.

Threats

The threat of the HMO was recognized as a major factor. To respond to it by developing a competing HMO, however, would be dependent on acceptance by the medical staff and patients. In general, the medical staff was opposed to a Kaiser model of HMO, but would accept an independent practice association (IPA) alternative. This would leave each free to have some fee-for-service and some capitation patients. Similarly, patients of the hospital expressed interest in an HMO as a device to control health insurance costs, but generally preferred to retain their own physicians. The results of this initial analysis indicated that Coastline should pursue the IPA idea further.

The threat of Morgan City's developing its own hospital was felt to be real, although the local HSA opposed the construction of any additional beds. After surveying the community to identify major concerns that prompted the desire for a hospital, Coastline concluded that the fear of an emergency and having to drive an excessive distance to the nearest hospital was the major factor, although community pride and economics also were considerations. As a result of this survey, Coastline decided to pursue the development of a freestanding emergency room satellite in Morgan City, staffed by contract physicians. Such a satellite could expand into a full-fledged source of primary care, ambulatory surgery, and even inpatient care in the long run. It also would serve as an attraction for signing up participants in the IPA, if that were developed.

Opportunities

The physical rehabilitation program seemed an attractive choice at first. Foreseeable increases in the number of aged would mean increased demand for rehabilitation from stroke and other infirmities associated with advanced age. On the other hand, the development of a successful program would depend on getting referrals from physicians throughout the area. Coastline is not viewed as a specialist hospital, and local physicians rarely if ever refer patients there unless they are on its medical staff. Moreover, the capital investment and staffing changes necessary for a rehabilitation program were enormous. The clincher lay in the discovery that Holy Family was actively pursuing the development of just such a program and already had begun recruiting a specialist in physical medicine and rehabilitation to direct it.

The possibility of merger with Holy Family was not considered a very positive option at first, whatever its feasibility. When preliminary contacts were made with Holy Family, however, it was discovered that it had some complementary interests. Holy Family was interested in concentrating more on its secondary/tertiary care programs but recognized the need for maintaining a solid base of primary level referrals. With a 25-bed rehabilitation unit being developed, it would lose the corresponding number of medical surgical beds and face increasing difficulty in placing all its patients. Following initial discussion, it was decided to pursue at least some shared planning to determine if future coordinated efforts would be worthwhile.

Discussion

The chief contribution of a marketing perspective to Coastline's approach was its focus on behavior and motivating factors. By identifying exactly whose behavior might be affected or would have to change if Coastline made a change, the hospital was able to examine its prospects from a more comprehensive perspective than if it had followed its preferences alone. It learned a lot about the motivations of its significant publics: patients, physicians, and competitors and how their behavior might change. As a result, it is able to concentrate its planning and marketing efforts on the specific persons whose behavior will determine their success.

DISCUSSION QUESTIONS

1. How would you describe the impact, behavior and cause results of a market audit of Coastline Community Hospital?
2. What problems, threats, and opportunities did the hospital not perceive or misinterpret?
3. What useful additional information could be included in this analysis?
4. If you were Coastal, what objectives would you pursue in the short run? What goals in the long run?
5. What strategies could you employ to accomplish these objectives:
   - whose behavior
   - would change to what
   - for what reasons
   - with what impact

Chapter 15

Passive Planning

This chapter is adapted from the case history of a hospital in New York State.[1] The names of actual hospitals and places involved were disguised in the original case description and are changed further here. While the particulars of the case in many facets are peculiar to New York State, the lessons are universal. Increasingly, the external environments created by planning, regulatory, and rate-setting agencies are becoming the most important consideration in marketing. The failure of Passive Hospital to realize the marketing implications of its intentions and aspirations provide a classic example of this development.

Figure 15-1 Hospitals Situated in the Area[2]

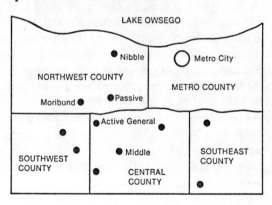

1. Brown, Jonathan B. *Facility Expansion and Facility Closure: Two Case Studies in Health Planning and Regulation from Rochester, New York.* Boston, Mass.: Harvard Center for Community Health and Medical Care, January 1978, pp. 7-55.
2. Except for Metro City, each dot represents one hospital.

Passive Hospital is a 150-bed, nonprofit community hospital located in Northwest County. (See Figure 15-1.) The county is predominantly rural, though its eastern, especially northeastern, areas serve as suburbs of Metro City, a metropolis of more than one million people, 30 miles northeast of Passive. While the town of Passive is the largest community in the county and enjoys general prosperity, the county seat is in Moribund, 12 miles to the west. The 25-bed Moribund Memorial Hospital began having trouble ten years ago when it failed state licensing inspection. Unable to obtain local or Hill-Burton funding to replace the old wooden frame building, the community of Moribund faced a crisis.

PROBLEMS ROOTED IN RIVALRY

Moribund and Passive are rivals of long standing. The annual high school football and basketball games invariably produce fights in the stands and intense feelings everywhere. Physicians at one hospital never practice or refer patients to the other; they rarely socialize and are barely polite to each other at medical society meetings. While Passive Hospital offers many specialized services, the physicians at Moribund invariably refer their patients all the way to Metro City in preference to Passive.

Other hospitals in the immediate area include Nibble Hospital (40 beds), 20 miles to the north, Active General Hospital (210 beds), ten miles southwest, and Middle Hospital (60 beds), 25 miles south. A number of other small hospitals dot the area, but do not figure prominently in this case.

Moribund was faced with a difficult choice: to build a minimum 50-bed facility in order to qualify for Hill-Burton funding and double the amount of capital risk or to close the hospital entirely. At the same time, Western County commissioners call for the building of a new 60-bed nursing home in the county. Moribund responds by suggesting a combination of 60 long-term care and 50 hospital beds to replace its existing facility. Passive insists that the new facility should be built next to its modern, 150-bed hospital. Passive suggests that it also would be willing to expand its facility by 50 beds to make up for the impending closure of Moribund Hospital and to accommodate expected population growth.

The local health planning agency that serves the five-county region acts favorably on Passive's suggestion, granting it a certificate of need to add 50 acute care beds. Moribund, with closure of its hospital inevitable, decides to press for a freestanding long-term care facility of 60 beds. The planning agency feels that location of LTC beds should be nearer to an acute facility, however, and requests that representatives of Moribund and Passive get together to see if they can come to agreement on a regional hospital/long-term care approach.

The first option discussed is to open up the board of trustees at Passive to a significant number of members representing Moribund. The bylaws of Passive, however, don't call for any board seats to be filled for another year, with only two openings even then. The medical staff of Passive will accept physicians at Moribund as courtesy or honorary members, but refuses to vote them full surgical privileges since they all lack surgical board eligibility or certification. Thus the effort to create a joint board or medical staff between Moribund and Passive comes to nothing.

The county commissioners line up with Moribund in its effort to have the new nursing home located there. Both the regional and state planning agencies, however, feel that location next to an acute care hospital is a critical factor and strongly encourage Passive to apply for a certificate of need to add extended care facility (ECF) beds. Passive acquiesces and submits an amended application calling for an addition of 50 acute care and 60 ECF beds. Despite the opposition of the county commissioners, Passive Hospital's application is approved and detailed planning and development follow.

Preliminary analysis calls for costs of $3.7 million for the entire project. Hill-Burton support is requested for $1.2 million and is approved. A fund-raising consultant agrees to raise at least $1 million, while Passive obtains commitments to loans for the balance. Analysis and projection of Passive's financial picture indicate that it can just manage the debt service that will result, provided it can maintain its prevailing level of 75 percent occupancy in the new acute facility, and 85 percent in the ECF.

When construction bids are opened, however, the lowest bid turns out to be $800,000 higher than the $3.7 million capital budget. The delays in development of final plans caused by the long-term care and Moribund closure issues coupled with rapid inflation in construction costs produced this unfortunate result. No further commitments from lending organizations are possible, so Passive has no choice but to take a hatchet to its equipment purchase plans and cut out all frills.

By paring the construction project to the bone, holding down on parking, office spaces, and ancillary space as well as equipment purchases, Passive manages to cut bids back to the original budget. The low bid is accepted and work is begun. By fast-tracking the construction (which also holds down costs), Passive is able to complete the project in two years. Parts of the new facility are opened in sequence, while renovations on the old proceed nearby.

Meanwhile, other developments have been taking place. Active General Hospital, which has been sitting on a certificate of need for 60 new beds issued some years earlier, decides to act on it. Because it is able to obtain financing through reserves, community fund drives, and loans with no Hill-Burton assistance, and despite substantially higher costs per bed, it is able to complete construction and open its new addition by the time Passive's new building is finished.

Population growth projected for the Passive area has failed to materialize. Major suburban sprawl has continued along the shore of the lake rather than south toward Passive. The decline in birth rates exacerbates the problem, which produces no net population growth in the Passive area for five years. The closing of a local textile mill with the loss of more than 500 jobs contributes to this result. State plans for highway construction that originally called for the new Interstate to pass close to Passive are shifted eight miles to the south and bypass the area completely.

The influx of patients from Moribund, anticipated after the closure of the hospital there, also fails to materialize. The physicians in that community were recruited to staff the emergency room at Active General, and patients from Moribund go either to Active or up to Metro City as before. The eight Moribund physicians are given full privileges at Active Hospital and use its new ambulatory surgery program extensively. To solidify its referral patterns from Moribund, Active develops a primary care satellite there, under its sponsorship but staffed by the former Moribund Hospital physicians.

With its brand new facility open for business, Passive discovers there isn't any. Declines in fertility leave its obstetrics unit operating at 45 percent occupancy, and pediatrics at 36 percent. Even its medical-surgical unit, which was severely overcrowded at 92 percent occupancy in the old facility, languishes at 64 percent occupancy in its expanded quarters. To make matters worse, the state has changed its systems of cost or charges reimbursement.

When Passive began its construction program, it could count on 72 percent of its patient days being paid by three third party sources: Blue Cross, Medicare, and Medicaid. All used the same reimbursement method: audited costs or charges, whichever is lower. While Passive felt constrained to keep its costs within reason, and still had to recover expenditures as best it could for the other 28 percent of patient days, this cost-based reimbursement meant it was never at too great a risk of overextension. If one service failed to operate in the black (e.g., obstetrics or pediatrics) the losses always could be recovered by services that made a profit (surgery, laboratory, x-ray, pharmacy).

By the time the new facility opened, however, a new system was in force. Costs of each service were examined carefully, and acceptable cost limits were calculated based on reasonable utilization levels. These were determined based on unit occupancy, as follows:

Medical-surgical beds	85 percent
Pediatrics	75 percent
Obstetrics	75 percent

Psychiatric	80 percent
ECF	90 percent

For example, if the total hospital's occupancy were required to be 80 percent, given its mix of beds, then costs would be calculated as if it accommodated the corresponding number of patient days (80 percent × bed supply × 365). If actual patient days were lower, costs per patient day would be higher than reimbursement levels. The hospital would collapse financially if it failed to meet occupancy expectations.

The option given to each hospital, faced with disaster because of foreseeable low occupancy, was to decertify enough of its beds so as to achieve the desired occupancy. If it projected only 66.7 percent occupancy of 120 beds (average daily census of 80 ÷ 120 = 66.7%) it could decertify 20 beds, resulting in 80 percent occupancy (80 ÷ 100). While the fixed costs of those 20 beds remained, the overall costs of operation for the hospital would be considered acceptable because it was achieving its desired occupancy.

Despite the many fallacies in this approach, it represented salvation for Passive Hospital. To qualify for the occupancy requirement, Passive was forced to decertify 55 beds, resulting in its becoming five beds smaller, on paper, than before the expansion. The state is threatening to increase its occupancy requirements in subsequent years, however, meaning that Passive may find itself diminishing in size still further in the future. Efforts are under way to regionalize obstetric and pediatric facilities as well. While Passive's 30-bed pediatric unit qualifies under national planning guidelines, its 900 obstetric deliveries do not. Closure of its obstetrics unit could result in loss of gynecology patients and pediatrics. Its once bright future has suddenly gone gray.

WHAT WENT WRONG?

The name given to Passive Hospital in this case denotes one major cause of its difficulties. Its basic approach was to foresee a future that looked very comfortable, and wait for it to happen, developing its facility so as to be ready for future admissions to drop into its lap. Such an approach is risky in any situation, and especially one in which there exists substantial competition, whose approach may be more active.

The beginning of all the trouble can be traced to how the closure of Moribund Hospital and the nursing home issue were handled. While the traditional rivalry between Passive and Moribund Hospitals and their communities were important factors, Passive was somewhat naive in assuming it would naturally inherit the patients let loose by the closure of Moribund Hospital.

The mistaken forecasts might have been beyond the power of anyone to foresee. Declines in fertility rates occurred over a long period of time, however, and impacts on pediatric (if not obstetric) census could be anticipated well in advance. Population growth patterns, while not easy to forecast in the long run, can be monitored through building permits, utility hook-ups, etc., to keep track of deviations from projections. Sudden changes in reimbursement policies may not be foreseeable via past trends, but in most cases are preceded by significant discussion periods.

In general, investments by health care organizations in anticipation of changes in population, behavior, or policy should be made in view of both the risks and the benefits involved. An investment of nearly $4 million, dependent on a series of independent, fortuitous developments, has enormous risks. Since any one of those developments (shift of patients from Moribund, population growth, continuation of cost reimbursement, steady fertility rates) could have produced trouble if it failed to come out as expected, Passive's depending on all four magnifies the extent of risk.

Coupled with the level of risk must be the seriousness of consequences. Passive Hospital acted on the belief that the most favorable outcomes would occur. Had it identified and anticipated the consequences of the least favorable, it might have acted differently. Its alternatives for less favorable developments included paring down or delaying expansion plans until it had better indications of what the future would be (population growth, fertility rates). Another choice would have been setting about to promote the probability of behavior more favorable to the anticipated outcomes (recruitment of Moribund physicians, lobbying for cost reimbursement).

By focusing on specific behaviors upon which its future was dependent, Passive Hospital might have been able to apply marketing techniques, research, and strategy to great benefit. Even intuitively it should have recognized that joint planning with the Moribund people should involve some quid pro quo. Unless it was willing to bend a little in such areas as board of trustees membership, medical staff privileges, and nursing home location, the effort at joint planning was doomed from the start.

Passive acted as if it had no competition, a dangerous approach even when it's true, but even more so when it isn't. Instead of assuming it would inherit all previous Moribund Hospital patients, it should have recognized the choices available to the physicians and the population involved. Despite its being in another county and slightly farther away, Active Hospital should have been identified as a significant competitive alternative. Had Passive examined its own offering in relation to what Active might offer, it would have realized in what a poor position it was putting itself. Active probably could have attracted the Moribund market for even less than it offered, considering the abysmal benefits Passive was willing to make available. The past history of patients' being referred past Passive to Metro City failed to warn Passive of the existing hostility, to say nothing of the added ill feelings generated by its failure to offer full board membership, staff privileges, and compromise on nursing home location.

As in any marketing situation in health care, ethical issues are raised in this case. It may be that sound professional reasons exist for limiting surgery privileges for general practitioners, or insisting on locating the nursing home next to an acute care hospital. However, the full consequences of such a stance must be anticipated and evaluated in judging its propriety. It might have been possible for surgical privileges for more routine operations to be granted the general practitioners at Moribund, rather than rejecting any granting of privileges, absent board eligibility or certification. Referral agreements and regular visits by medical staff might have retained most of the quality advantages relative to location of the nursing home while still permitting Moribund to retain a source of community pride.

Passive saw itself as the natural choice to serve as the regional hospital center for Northwest County. It was lulled into believing the inevitability of this development by plans published by the regional planning agency. This agency employed traditional Hill-Burton methods that identified service populations by county. From the planning agencies' viewpoint, all residents of Northwest County did and would use hospitals in that county. That this was not true should have been apparent from the extremely high apparent use rates calculated for Metro City vs. low rates for the surrounding counties. This phenomenon commonly results from ignoring patient travel and dividing all patient days in an area by the population of that area, despite large numbers of persons who may go elsewhere or come in from elsewhere for care.

This inflow/outflow reality tends to produce exaggerated use rates in all urban areas and understated rates in rural. The Hill-Burton method traditionally assumes also that use rates won't change. In this case, Utilization Review, PSRO, and cost containment efforts, coupled with declining fertility rates, produced significant drops in use rates. This resulted from an increase in ambulatory surgery as opposed to inpatient (an increase promoted by hospitals other than Passive) and a general decline in length of stay.

Moreover, the patterns of patient travel were by no means limited by county boundaries. Passive expected to inherit the patients from Moribund because they were in the same county. It had similar expectations for patients from Nibble, which had been targeted for closure but actually had expanded and rebuilt as population growth along the lake shore built up its census. The natural pattern of travel from Nibble probably would have been to Metro City anyway, just as the pattern from Moribund ended up toward Active Hospital.

Passive might have diminished or even prevented the loss of the Moribund market through a number of strategies. Even after alienating the Moribund medical staff, there existed the possibility of developing an ambulatory care satellite in Moribund sponsored by Passive. By offering care within the community, such a program might have competed very effectively with Active Hospital's programs. Passive's policy of refusing to perform abortions also tended to alienate some physicians and many prospective patients, although changing it could have had mixed results.

Passive Hospital failed to recognize that if a truly regional system were to develop in the area, Active Hospital was in a far better position to serve as the referral center than Passive. Active is more centrally located among the hospitals that don't naturally refer toward Metro City, it is larger, and at least as well-staffed and well-equipped. Passive can be considered a center (see Figure 15-1) only if the existence of Metro City's hospitals is ignored. By failing to see the regional idea from an objective viewpoint, Passive missed the reality that Active had more to gain than it did.

The decision by Passive to cut equipment and amenities to the bone, however forced by financial realities, was unfortunate. Internally, it may have been justifiable, once a commitment to the expansion was made. In terms of marketing, however, it left the institution in a seriously inferior competitive position relative to Active. With Active's ability to obtain full funding for a first-class new institution, Passive's market position as the most modern, fully equipped hospital in the region disappeared.

Recognizing the competition from Active Hospital, Passive might have begun an attempt to develop a coordinated relationship, reserving some distinct role in a regional system for itself while yielding on services where Active's competitive edge was substantial. Passive failed even to consider what Active might do, despite knowing that Active retained certificate-of-need permission to construct a new facility. Active laid its groundwork first by recruiting the medical staff from Moribund and ensuring full funding for a first-class project rather than gambling. While both Passive and Active delayed construction, incurring inflationary increases in cost, Active used the delay to promote the success of its venture while Passive was bogged down in a fight over the nursing facility.

In effect, Active Hospital employed a marketing strategy, whether consciously or not, to increase the likelihood that its project would turn out successfully. It identified what behaviors its success was dependent on or could be increased by the inheritance of Moribund Hospital's medical staff and patients. It avidly recruited the medical staff through arranging for its members to cover the emergency room, giving them a free work space and an on-site tie to the hospital. By offering them full staff privileges, Active destroyed any likelihood that the physicians would join Passive's staff. The ambulatory surgery center arrangement was set up so that Moribund's physicians would concentrate on simple surgery, avoiding much of the concern over their lack of training.

Active did benefit somewhat from the fact that the Interstate highway was built closer to it than to Passive. However, by waiting until construction of the highway and its location were assured, it avoided a gamble on the subject. It also was not gambling on population growth in its direction but designed its project based on the population already available. While it did not foresee the change in reimbursement, it was aware that as costs for health care rose at alarming rates following the passage of Medicare/Medicaid, the cost-based system couldn't last forever. Given the 20- to 30-year expected life of a hospital facility, it decided to plan for high occupancy rather than mere size. Moreover, rather than merely forecasting its future census, it did something about it.

The choice of forecasting vs. doing something about the future is a recurring option in health services development. Given the uncertainty of any such effort, there always is a risk in relying on forecasts, even if developed by prominent governmental agencies. Besides, forecasts of population growth don't always translate into population behavior. New arrivals are least likely to adopt prevailing behavior patterns and are most receptive to new sources and programs of health care delivery. If new arrivals move from only a few miles away, however, they probably will retain their previous sources of care and not adopt the local system.

The options available to physicians traditionally have constituted a buyers' market. Hospitals always have had to compete with each other in recruiting medical staff, and rural hospitals traditionally have been at a disadvantage. There are signs this situation is changing, although rural hospitals may be the last to notice it. As the ratio of physicians to population continues to increase (doubling between 1950 and 2000) while the number of hospitals actually diminishes, and if excess bed capacity is reduced, a new market situation may result.

If it shifts from a buyers' to a sellers' market, hospitals may be able to behave like Passive Hospital in this case, requiring any physician wishing to join their staffs to conform to strict requirements. The prices hospitals in rural areas now charge (committee meetings, medical record keeping, emergency room coverage) may be increased significantly. The product may be tilted a little more away from being the workshop offering whatever tools the physicians demand. As hospitals become part of larger regional systems, the ability of physicians to threaten to take their patients elsewhere becomes a less and less credible alternative.

What long-run effects such a shift might have can only be speculated upon at this point. Passive Hospital's stance in relation to Moribund physicians clearly was premature. Moreover, acting as if you're the seller in a sellers' market always runs the risk of alienating buyers toward future shifts in the market, or toward competitors who still prefer courting customers. Effective market relationships have to produce acceptable cost/benefit or product/price trades for both parties involved, or they won't endure long.

The ethical aspects of marketing were clearly in evidence in this case, although Passive Hospital paid for its self-righteous professionalism in terms of the outcome. Whether the obligation of individual providers and organizations is toward upholding rigid standards or optimizing total outcomes in their decisions is a choice each of us has to make. Like any organization, health care delivery institutions have to survive in order to accomplish anything, yet survival at the expense of professional ethics may not be a fair exchange.

Passive's largest single mistake in this case was focusing its attention on a single important but insufficient factor in the market—the planning agency. As far as this regulatory factor was concerned, Passive did everything right. The hospital responded only to needs identified by the planning organization, and planned developments in strict accord with published plan documents and policies on regionalization. Clearly, maintaining effective relations with regulatory agencies is an ever-present necessity for health care organizations, but it isn't the only necessity. By failing to recognize how much its success depended on the behavior of other organizations, Passive failed either to assess the extent and impact of its risks or to do anything about reducing them.

Passive made the blunder of assuming that what the state and regional planning agencies identified as desirable—the closure of small hospitals and development of a regional system focused on Passive—would necessarily come true. Where it felt it could count on the closure of Nibble and even Middle Hospital to enhance its own market position, only the Moribund facility actually did close. Moreover, while the official planning agencies ceded the Moribund and Nibble markets to Passive, Nibble probably wouldn't have adhered to the plan, and Moribund didn't.

Given the difficulties planning agencies have in implementing their often commendable ideals, Passive certainly was overoptimistic in its expectations. The hospital would have been far better off doing some research on population behavior and attitudes rather than swallowing the assumptions contained in the regional plan. Passive would have done better to approach the Moribund physicians as valued potential customers rather than as supplicants, and recruit them rather than self-righteously stipulate conditions under which they would be allowed to join the medical staff. This preferred approach is justified in any market situation, but especially so where competition exists or might develop.

The series of blunders Passive Hospital committed represent almost a classic example of nonmarketing and its subsequent failure. It would seem almost absurd to describe such a case even as an extreme cartoon of the dangers of nonmarketing, were it not for the fact that the case is based on fact. While the particulars in some instances have been changed to protect confidentiality and enhance learning, the essence of the hospital's approach was left intact. Certainly all those who read this will recognize, in hindsight, the absurdity of the hospital's approach, but the hospital failed to appreciate it in foresight.

It is to be hoped that we can learn from mistakes, both our own and those of others. There is no way of guaranteeing that had Passive Hospital adopted a marketing approach, it would have been able to fill its new facility. Instead, a good market research effort might have pointed out merely the futility of expansion. Every health care organization has the same choice in market positioning: molding itself to meet the market, or influencing the market to fit its desires and capabilities. The first requires effective research and sensitivity; the second, charismatic salesmanship. Neither extreme is recommended as a standard approach. Effective compromises are likely to be necessary and appropriate in most instances. The decision is up to you.

*   *   *

Grateful acknowledgment is hereby made to Jonathan B. Brown, M.P.P., the author of the case history upon which this case is based. While the adaptation is strictly the responsibility of this book's author, Brown's permission and comments in allowing the case to be included here were accepted with delight. The real story upon which the case was based includes other lessons, more thoroughly documented in the original work cited at the beginning of this chapter. That it provides so many useful lessons in a marketing text testifies to the comprehensive, insightful description provided by Brown and to the overlap between effective planning and effective marketing.

Chapter 16

Hospital Marketing: Promotion

Coast Community Hospital (CCH) is a 150-bed acute care, proprietary hospital operated by a large hospital chain. It is a fully equipped, modern facility on the city line between two coastal cities, Beachville and Sandy Point. Each city has a population of about 50,000 year-round, but there is a large influx of tourists in the summer because of the seashore location. The hospital offers an above-average type of medical-surgical services but no obstetrics or radiation therapy. The outpatient service is large and is available to all local physicians.

Adjacent to CCH is a physicians' office building constructed four years before the hospital was opened. At the time the hospital was completed the medical office building was occupied only partially. All but three of the 15 physicians in the building were specialists. A strong polarization of civic pride and blind loyalty between Beachville and Sandy Point permeates the medical and hospital referral patterns and it was unthinkable for patterns to cross city lines. When the new hospital appeared on the boundary line, both cities viewed it with suspicion since it could line up with either one and certainly not with both. What a challenge: to be successful, Coast Community would have to attract referrals from both sides.

There are three other hospitals in the area. The 300-bed Beachville Memorial and the 200-bed Sandy Point Memorial are local government-owned, full-service hospitals with active emergency rooms. These two hospitals have been serving their respective cities for the last 15 to 20 years. Across the street from Beachville Memorial is the 100-bed Park Central Hospital, a proprietary institution recently sold by its physician owners to a small but growing hospital chain. The major market segments of interest to Coast Community are served by the three existing hospitals. Of the three, only Park Central is seeking additional physicians and patients aggressively. Chronic underfunding and a relatively stable occupancy keep the two civic hospitals from actively seeking more patients.

RESEARCH

The Coast Community Hospital opened in 1976 with moderate initial success due to the support of the physicians in the adjacent office building. Beginning in 1977, intensive market research efforts were begun to identify key demographic segments, market shares from those segments, and realistic targets, and to develop responsive strategies for census building. Simple patient origin statistics identified existing markets and, after a rough percentage of market share was calculated, certain areas were targeted to be tapped for more admissions. Initial analysis indicated that several geographic areas inland from the beach were producing few admissions to Coast Community, despite the fact that it was the closest health care facility. Analysis and mapping of physicians' offices and residences indicated that few physicians practiced in these residential, semirural areas. An extensive telephone interview survey revealed that the residents either never had established a family physician relationship or were traveling to primary care physicians' offices near the Beachville and Sandy Point hospitals and were receiving care at those facilities.

The physician residence and office locater map also illustrated which physicians, by specialty, were residing or practicing closer to Coast Community than the three competitor hospitals but had not applied to CCH for staff membership. This study also was valuable in identifying the distribution of specialists and primary care providers and in analyzing their relationships to each other and to the hospitals they utilized. Voids in the patterns and/or shortages of certain specialists and services were labeled easily. Phone and face-to-face interviews with key physicians were accomplished and valuable data were gathered on the attitudes, preferences, needs, and practice problems of those in the target areas. Physicians were asked to comment from their own perspective and to report their colleagues' opinions. The physicians' perception of their associates' opinions was especially interesting, revealing, and helpful.

Patients admitted to Coast Community were surveyed twice during their exposure to the new hospital. One questionnaire was completed during the admitting procedure. Patients were asked whether they or their physician chose Coast Community, why they chose it (if CCH was their choice), or whether they would have preferred another facility (if CCH was their physician's choice). "Why" questions followed each response to determine the relative level of accurate knowledge about CCH. One question was designed to find out how the patient first heard about CCH (i.e., media, friends, previous admission, etc.). The second questionnaire was completed at or after discharge and was designed to test the level of satisfaction with the services provided.

Competitors were examined to determine their strengths and weaknesses, the existence of vacant or partly satisfied actual and psychological market positions, and styles of practice. They obviously enjoyed community identification, were saddled with a particular reputation, and held the loyalty of their older staff physicians. They tended to be cold, formal, efficient, and impersonal toward patients through autocratic, heavily structured policies regarding visitors, physicians, and personal patient habits. This opened the potential of appealing to younger and newly established physicians who could share in building their own medical staffs rather than competing with the power structures entrenched at the older hospitals. It also created the possibility of reaching patients with a friendly, casual, humanistic, open institutional personality.

MARKET OBJECTIVES

Coast Community defined its market objectives in terms of physicians and patients since its initial analysis showed that patients frequently shared the decision on which hospital they would be admitted to and often adamantly insisted on the only one they would use. Therefore, the potential patient market was separated into three groups:

1. prior or current patients—those engaged with the physicians in the medical office building and who had been admitted to or utilized outpatient services from CCH

2. local residents who were not patients—those who could be made aware of and interested in what Coast Community had to offer

3. nonresidents—those who had moved to the area recently or who were tourists and were making a choice of which hospital to use for specific services such as emergency care

Physician markets were separated into three segments also:

1. active physicians—those on the staff at CCH whose activity and loyalty were to be increased and solidified (mostly specialists)

2. inactive physicians—those not on the staff at CCH but whose referrals or staff applications could be attracted (mostly primary care)

3. needed physicians—those individuals who could be recruited into the area by CCH to set up practice and support CCH primarily.

PATIENT STRATEGIES

Separate though complementary strategies were designed and implemented for the three patient markets. Current patients were impressed, purposefully, with warm, human concern and casual policies. Patients were treated as "customers" and their personal needs as human beings were met along with their medical needs. Patients could not help but express their positive impressions to CCH staff members and these were recorded and printed in a monthly newsletter. This strategy served two important purposes: (1) It focused the attention of CCH staff members on patient attitudes and the importance of satisfaction. (2) It disseminated positive patient attitudes toward the hospital to other local residents.

As specific departments and individual staff members were singled out by patient praise, a friendly spirit of competition developed in the organization. Nursing units, for example, began to pride themselves and vie for producing greater positive impressions with their patients. Individual employees saw their attitudes reflected in the patients' comments and received recognition for pleasing customers. This further imprinted the attitude that personal, as well as medical, care were important. The increasing frequency of positive comments from satisfied patients, the uplifted employee morale, and a steadily rising census all attested to the success of this strategy.

This attitude would not have been possible without the constant attempt to identify, accept, and respond to patients' human needs and wants wherever reasonable. Visiting hours were open, rules were liberal and situational, healthy children were allowed to visit loved ones, special dietary needs were supplied, and the maintenance of the warmth of the family unit while one member was hospitalized was encouraged. All this was under the direction of the physician and subject to his order. Satisfied patients caused skeptical physicians to support the whole strategy and this increased and solidified their activity.

This strategy was supported by a novel "customer awareness" seminar for all employees based on airline stewardess training and aimed at sensitizing personnel to be aware of and responsive to patient and family needs. A patient care representative or ombudsman encouraged patient comments, coordinated the satisfaction of patient or family needs, and pursued inevitable complaints. Comments from customers attested to the feeling that, if you must be in a hospital, Coast Community was the place to be since it was nicer than most hotels and certainly better than the typical, stereotyped "hospital service."

Recognizing that emergency service represented a substantial source of inpatients, CCH developed a strategy to compete with the existing emergency rooms at the other hospitals. Research revealed the others offered a physician-on-duty from evening until morning and relied on a rotating call schedule during the day. Their reputation was one of making patients wait for the physician and for service. Upon opening, Coast Community offered 24-hour onduty physicians and stressed this coverage in the publicity campaigns. Indications from local industry reflected dissatisfaction with the other hospitals' promptness and accuracy in handling on-the-job injuries. CCH developed and hand-distributed an emergency kit to hundreds of retail businesses and heavy industrial concerns in a geographical area closer to Coast Community than to the other hospitals. This kit contained:

- a standard first aid kit with a map of the location of CCH in relation to the business imprinted on the cover

- "Emergency Data Wallet Cards" with a map on one side and space for pertinent medical information on the other, to be distributed to all employees and family members

- a poison antidote medicine chest chart

- a cardio-pulmonary resuscitation (CPR) technique wall chart

- brochures describing Coast Community's emergency room

- a display map with "you are here" feature showing the most direct route to the closest emergency room at CCH for posting in each place of business

- emergency care phone stickers

These informational and educational devices provided the essential cue for swaying unpredictable choices regarding source of care—a constant reminder designed to be the first thing an individual might see when an emergency arose and providing a readily available source of medical information to persons forced to cope with the emergency.

Potential new patients—those local residents unaware of Coast Community—were approached through a number of educational and promotional strategies. The intent of the market strategy was to educate and inform by providing helpful medical knowledge and to imprint the Coast Community name and logo by associating the source of the help with the particular hospital. This was accomplished in two ways: (1) a medical information tape library with 300 subjects accessible through the telephone and (2) the sponsorship of five 30-second television spots each week on a local station. The taped medical information system was Tel Med, professionally prepared and marketed nationally by a California-based corporation. Coast Community distributed thousands of brochures listing the topics and phone number through the public school system, racks in public places, clubs, groups, etc. Each caller was greeted by the phrase, "Coast Community Tel Med, may I help you?" and each tape concluded with the phrase, "This has been another community service of Coast Community Hospital." The television spots were produced inexpensively by the local station in return for guaranteed paid time. Each "Health Hint" began with the logo and name of the hospital and concluded with the hospital name. The TV spots were public education providing helpful information on what to do if a child swallowed poison, how to treat simple cuts and burns, what to do for jellyfish stings and insect bites, etc. This market strategy reached hundreds of potential new patients each day and tied helpful, caring health information to the name of the provider of this information: Coast Community Hospital.

Other strategies involved free public service announcements over local radio stations on a daily basis. These publicized the many health education services, classes, tours, etc., provided by the hospital.

In addition to the media approach, hundreds of brochures were made available to anyone interested in a particular topic. The hospital ordered free brochures from all special interest societies (i.e., American Heart, Diabetes, Cancer, Kidney, etc.) and after overstamping with the name and logo, provided them free to all through various outlets.

Brochures were helpful in this strategy, but they did not get the potential patient physically into the facility. To accomplish this, CCH began to conduct tours for schools, Scouts, clubs, etc., and invited the public into the hospital for free blood pressure screening, free blood typing, and free diabetes and kidney disease testing. The hospital's conference rooms were full of potential patients almost every night as various groups held their meetings. If space was available, no organization was turned away and thus many individuals became familiar with and grateful to the hospital. All this exposure did impose some administrative and maintenance costs, but it resulted in a very positive local image in a short time and impacted the public in both Beachville and Sandy Point equally and simultaneously.

Tourists and new residents were approached through such mechanisms as phone book covers and real estate booklets. Placards describing the location of the hospital and the services available were placed in shopping centers, motels, gas stations, and yacht clubs. The availability of 24-hour emergency services was prominently featured. City and seashore maps were imprinted with the name of the hospital and its central location obviously marked. The maps, together with a list of emergency telephone numbers (including the hospital's poison information hotline, Tel Med tape library, and emergency room contact numbers) were distributed to new arrivals via the various Welcome Wagon services.

Community-based screening services for hypertension, diabetes, and kidney disease were offered periodically in shopping centers and public schools. Positive results were communicated to the family physician if reported by screened residents; or the resident was directed to see a physician and given a preprinted card with the names and phone numbers of ten physicians who had consented to see screened patients requiring care. All physicians on the card were on staff at Coast Community, but some practiced primarily at another hospital. Follow-up study showed that, in general, patients referred to physicians by a screening program were admitted, if necessary, to the referral source. Protection of the reciprocal nature of the referral pattern by the physician seemed to be a natural physician reflex, even if the referral source was a hospital.

As the image of health information was maintained by the aggressive market strategy, the hospital was called on to provide an information service to anyone wishing to select a physician. In this situation, no attempt was made to restrict choice to only those physicians on CCH's staff since this would have irritated certain members of the medical community and created serious professional opposition to the solicitation of patients. The goodwill generated resulted in a substantial number of persons seeking Coast Community as a source of care and contacting physicians at the nearby medical office complex.

PHYSICIAN STRATEGIES

Physician strategies also varied for the different segments. While intense rivalry and polarization of loyalties existed between the two communities and their medical supports, CCH had to promote and encourage joint staff membership. This crossover was accomplished through two primary programs: (1) development of needed specialized services, and (2) the qualification of the hospital as an institution accredited for continuing medical education. Through long- and short-range planning and goal setting, CCH embarked on the periodic development of new services unique to the area, services for which the local physicians would look to CCH. Some of these included highly specialized lab tests, biplane angiography, alcohol rehabilitation, stress testing and 24-hour EKG scanning, hyperalimentation, blood cell washing, peripheral vascular diagnostic testing, endoscopy laboratory, minisurgery (one-day), and pulmonary function testing. Each service was unavailable elsewhere, represented the state of the art in equipment, and was introduced with informational brochure mailings to the physicians and with a public news conference.

Recognizing the increasing importance of organized continuing educational requirements to specialty boards, a strategy was designed to make Coast Community the only hospital in the area able to grant CME Category 1 credit for attendance at the monthly scientific meetings. Accreditation was applied for and granted by the American Medical Association in 1978. Physicians on the CCH staff could gather hours of continuing medical education (CME) credit just for attendance at regular staff scientific meetings and by participating in quarterly weekend seminars sponsored by the hospital. CCH became a significant force to be reckoned with as physicians pressured the administration and staff officers at the other hospitals to provide similar services for their staffs. Many outside physicians broke the geographic barrier and applied for staff membership just to avail themselves of the education programs and credits. Admission of patients followed the broken barrier, since these physicians now felt more comfortable with the "enemy."

When patients arrived in the emergency room, every effort was made to identify their family physicians and involve them in the case. Even where admission was not required, a report of the visit, treatment, and referral was sent to the patient's physician with the patient's permission.

Many strategies used by Coast Community were classic demonstrations of marketing as an exchange of benefits. The hospital executive director learned of a local physician not on the staff who was searching for someone to join him in practice. The director offered the services of the hospital's parent company physician recruiter. This gesture resulted in locating a partner. Both physicians now send a significant number of patients to Coast Community, though they have not switched active medical staff membership. Because the hospital shared its capability to recruit and therefore provided a significant benefit to the local physician, the physician simply returned the favor.

The number of referrals from medical staff members at the two civic hospitals increased steadily after Coast Community opened, but few physicians switched a majority of their practice. Such switches were not accepted well by the medical communities, and families of physicians who switched were likely to be ostracized by their peers and social groups. Even referrals to CCH for services potentially available at one of the civic hospitals were likely to be considered traitorous. However, despite this intense feeling, Coast Community was being viewed increasingly as an acceptable alternative, rather than a competitor.

Physicians on the medical staff were augmented in two ways. Additional specialists were attracted to the medical building next door, and their admissions to CCH followed automatically. Primary care physicians also were recruited to shore up the fragile referral base in the adjoining cities. Monthly scientific dinner meetings featured cocktails and prime rib buffet with the important CME credit-earning programs. Semiannual dinner dance parties for the staff physicians and spouses also demonstrated how highly CCH regarded physicians.

Many of the potential patient information and education programs also helped the local physicians. The poison information hotline and Tel Med tape information systems provided a constant influx of patients into the private offices for care. The emergency room provided a backup for the staff physicians after hours since the onduty emergency room physician could assess the patient condition and admit for the attending physician. This ER strategy was designed to augment and not threaten the active physician since the ER staff could not be engaged in practice outside the hospital. This feature promoted excellent staff relations.

In response to research results illustrating the lack of adequate physician offices providing primary care in the semirural area inland from Coast Community and the obvious lack of admissions from that sector, CCH developed two primary care satellite offices. One was in a small convenience store center in the middle of a growing residential area. The other was in a major shopping center among 30 or 40 busy commercial stores and entertainment businesses. Both featured convenient parking and location. Both soon recorded many admissions that would not have occurred otherwise. Preadmission testing services were made available at these locations as well as at the physicians' office building near the hospital for the convenience of patients and physicians.

Special efforts were made to attract and accommodate emergency referrals. Onduty sleeping facilities were set up for ambulance drivers at the hospital and patch phone lines to the dispatch stations were provided. The hospital cafeteria was opened around the clock to support emergency crews, police, physicians, and families of patients, as well as night shift hospital employees. More than 50,000 Emergency Data Wallet Cards were distributed to residents in the area. These simple but effective data cards stimulated the card carriers to identify with Coast Community. A number of large companies in the area were contacted at a luncheon and their representatives agreed to provide employees who were covered under a company health insurance policy with a special identification card from Coast Community. The card was designated "HCDR" or "Health Care Data Registry" and, after completing an identification document, the employee was issued an embossed plastic card for use when seeking service at CCH. The card did not directly entitle the individual to a line of credit, but cued the hospital admitting personnel that the person was employed and covered by group insurance. The information on the card was imprinted on various forms used for outpatient or emergency services and greatly speeded identification procedures.

RESULTS

These marketing strategies were employed incrementally after the hospital opened. The results as of this writing have been modest, but very encouraging. Hospital occupancy has risen steadily, while it has declined elsewhere in the area. A sample of two months' census over a three-year period illustrates this growth in percentage of occupancy:

August 1976	48.3	September 1976	51.6
August 1977	68.4	September 1977	67.3
August 1978	77.6	September 1978	78.5

The hospital had been breaking even financially for a year, and anticipated continuing significant improvement. Active competition from Park Central still was intense, especially under its new owners, and the negative feelings among many associated with the civic hospitals still persisted. Negative comments by some physicians in the area always could be expected, including some from those on the active staff at Coast Community. Most related to the high profile of CCH and what some considered the "tackiness" or "inappropriateness" of some promotional efforts. The steady growth, increased medical staff membership, and positive patient feedback tended to keep such objections to a minimum.

The emergency room saw rapidly increasing numbers of patients, especially following distribution of the emergency kits to local businesses. January volume in 1977 was 498 visits. This frequency increased to 573 in 1978 and 703 in 1979. While significant variations are characteristic from month to month in any emergency room, each month in 1978 was higher than the corresponding month in 1977 and the average number of visits per month in each year showed a 30 percent increase. A reliable and significant proportion of inpatient admissions came through the emergency room, so census benefited, as did laboratory and radiology volume. The fact that such significant gains in emergency room visits occurred while Coast Community's own efforts increased the availability of primary care physicians made it all the more remarkable.

The hospital's total medical staff membership at the opening was 28 physicians who responded to an initial mailing of 114 applications to prospective members in the area. This number increased to 52 in 1978 and 79 physicians in 1979. It is interesting to note that in 1977, 93 percent of the patients admitted were under the care of physicians in the adjacent medical office building and by 1979 this percentage had decreased to 82 percent, showing a significant amount of outside support from local physicians.

DISCUSSION

Since Coast Community did not survey consumer attitudes before it began its marketing efforts, there was no "before" picture to use in comparing current attitudes. There certainly was some face validity to presuming that promotional efforts and marketing strategies succeeded in changing behavior, but it was impossible to discern which specific efforts were successes or whether others were counterproductive. Patient satisfaction levels had been monitored since 1977, and the hospital continued to impress and satisfy its customers. The attitudes of the medical staff members were monitored each year by a corporate program of the parent company and no obvious positive change had been identified, although referrals steadily increased.

This was neither a negative nor a surprising finding. Satisfaction levels of physicians are a function of how well their expectations are met. Over time, such expectations are likely to rise, especially as they tend to be fulfilled. Satisfying physicians one year causes their expectations to rise, so that even if a hospital does better in an absolute sense, it may not have "improved" according to the changing physician expectations. Unfortunately, our own standards or expectations do tend to rise as they are met; it is only frustration that causes them to stand still or even drop. Since the essential behavior has changed positively, the disappointing attitude survey results cannot be viewed with alarm.

If satisfaction levels were to drop, and the promises of alternative behavior seem more attractive, then behavioral change might follow and do some damage. It is the combination of dissatisfaction with current arrangements and the emergence of an apparently superior alternative that tends to change behavior, with the emphasis generally on the latter factor. This is why it is useful to attempt to link attitudes with behavior rather than merely presume a direct relationship exists.

Coast Community by no means relied on promotional marketing strategies to increase census and overcome civic polarization. It recognized that communication was only partially effective in changing behavior. The strategies developed were intended to actually improve the product (i.e., service and the place and style of making that service available). Many strategies reduced the price of doing business with CCH. In the marketplace, Coast Community could not rely on persuasion alone. The emphasis on pleasing patients, on treating them as human beings and as valued customers rather than as bodies filling beds and increasing revenues, was clearly a product improvement. Convenient visiting policies and hours, food selection, room arrangements, inpatient education, and ID medical data cards all enhanced the benefit vs. cost of being one of Coast Community's customers.

Similarly, many distinct advantages were afforded the physicians on CCH's staff. Assistance with initial practice set up, both advisory and financial, were available to newly recruited physicians, medical office space was close to the hospital, the ER night call services prevented the necessity of coming to the hospital to see a patient at night, and the CME credits were awarded for attendance at scientific staff meetings and hospital seminars. These strategies offered important benefits to physicians with patients at Coast Community.

In recruiting new medical staff, the ready referral to specialists was helpful in attracting primary care physicians. Conversely, the growing number of primary care physicians, including those in the strategically placed satellite centers, helped attract specialists. Each offered to the others prospects of both economic and professional advantages. Coast Community's marketing strategies recognized and embraced the synergistic interdependence of specialists, primary care physicians, and the hospital's organized medical staff.

The only market Coast Community overlooked was the three other hospitals themselves. While recruiting physicians and attracting admissions placed CCH in direct competition with the three, it should not automatically have precluded cooperation. There might be opportunities for shared service or ways to identify the optimum market position for CCH by working with the three rather than against them. Even if only one of the three could become an ally, there were possible advantages, although rivalry and competition were especially fierce in this specific area.

The lack of cooperation and coordination promised future difficulties with the local planning and regulatory agencies. Coast Community managed to get its program and facility going against great odds, but it earned the resentment of the state planning agency and might have trouble in the future. CCH tends to be viewed as overly entrepreneurial, not only because it is one of the few for-profit hospitals in the state but because of its highly visible marketing activities.

Even though its costs are comparable to the other facilities, except that it pays taxes, it is accused of "skimming" the best-paying patients and high-revenue services rather than being open to anyone without regard for financial willingness or ability to pay for services provided. What is effective market segmentation (no OB care, suburban location, preadmission financial screening on elective admissions, specialty care) from one perspective (the hospital's) can be viewed as exploitative skimming from another (the planning agency's).

The only way to avoid charges of skimming is to arrive at a market position either in direct response to local planning priorities or in concert with other institutions. Whether either would have been possible in this particular situation is open to question. They are alternatives worth considering in most circumstances. Adversary relationships with planning agencies and regulatory bodies are likely to be at least an inconvenience to most hospitals, but in some situations they can be crippling. Market analysis and strategy design can help avoid negative relationships in many instances, but often the price of avoidance is compromising what the institution prefers to do.

The promotional/educational communications strategies used in this case had definite legitimate public value. The same messages that promoted and imprinted the identity and image of the hospital provided useful information and education to the public. This is the essence of the effective promotion campaign—arranging the messages so that people in general, as well as the organization, specifically benefit from each communication. None of the messages were puffery, the comparative advertising specifically criticized by the American Hospital Association Guidelines on Advertising.

Targets for communications were segmented specifically so that concentrated efforts could be directed properly, but general strategies and necessary overlap were not ignored. The internal newsletters were distributed for maximum exposure, not only to employees but to patients, visitors, and potential patients so all could be impressed by emphasis on positive patient experiences. Messages intended for permanent residents also were received by new arrivals and tourists via radio, television, and newspaper. While the nature and focus of such messages may have been narrow, the potential effects and impacts were much wider.

One concern that must remain unanswered is the potential negative side effects of communications strategies. It probably did appear "unseemly" for Coast Community to advertise so blatantly when no other health care provider had tried anything like it before and has not tried anything like it since. CCH's obvious and aggressive efforts no doubt aroused the ire of local hospitals and of some physicians. This may limit any future attempt to cooperate or it simply may be the unavoidable price for penetrating a conservative marketplace with effective marketing strategies.

Chapter 17

A Primary Care Center Disaster

The entry of hospitals into the primary care market has been a recent but burgeoning development throughout the United States. Literally hundreds of hospitals have developed onsite or satellite primary care centers; many operate more than one. By and large, judging from the literature, such developments have been successful. Whether this is due to well-designed and well-executed programs, the natural potential of the market, or the reluctance of hospitals to write about their failures is not clear. Ambulatory care in general, and primary care in particular, have been touted as the best bet for future hospital development.

It often is true that we accept our successes uncritically, assuming they demonstrate our moral or technical superiority; we rarely learn much from them. Our failures are more likely to be learning experiences; unfortunately, we rarely communicate them to others. A team of professionals at the University of Kentucky is virtually unique in that it participated in and described for others to read an instructional failure in primary care development. The team learned much from the experience and did the field an enormous service by describing it in a published article.[1]

The author makes grateful acknowledgment of the contribution made by the four authors in reminding us what problems can arise if we fail to employ an effective marketing approach. The case combines insights based on their experience plus that of the author in a series of primary care development situations. It is hoped that the negative consequences of not employing effective marketing concepts and techniques will provide useful insights to readers.

---

1. Cowen, David L., M.D.; Hochstrasser, Donald L., Ph.D., M.P.H.; Fredericks, Carl, M.D., and Payne, John, M.D., M.P.H. "Problems in the Development of a Rural Primary Care Center." *Journal of Community Health* 2:1, Fall 1976, pp. 52-59.

THE CASE IN A POOR RURAL SETTING

Rural County is a fairly typical rural community of roughly 10,000 persons, dependent on agriculture and fishing, both of which are seasonal and neither providing long-term nor widespread prosperity. Based on a survey of the community, its health status is abnormally low and the use of health services unusually high. It has an aged population more than twice as large proportionately as the national average. Unemployment varies seasonally but averages 18 percent. More than 50 percent of the population lives below the national poverty index.

Work losses due to illness were reported as an average of 12.8 days per worker per year, more than double the national rate. Illness days per person per year were 32.6, almost exactly double the national average. Hospital admission rates were .384 per thousand population, almost two and a half times the national rate, while average length of stay was 11.2 days, almost four days higher than the U.S. average. While age adjustment reduces some of the apparent discrepancy, even on an age-adjusted basis, hospital use rates of 4,300 patient days per thousand are more than double what would be expected.

Such data clearly suggested the need for a radically new approach to health care delivery. National policy concerns with high levels of hospital utilization and high health care costs indicated the need for greater emphasis on prevention and ambulatory care. The physician serving Rural County was 70 years old. While loved, honored, and respected by the community, he was not able to keep up with its health care demands, nor with the realities of modern health care delivery. National Health Service Corps physicians moved to Rural County periodically but none stayed. The local hospital, despite Hill-Burton and community support, never was sufficient to attract an adequate supply of physicians. The nearest alternative sources of care were 37 miles away.

While the doctor was past retirement age, he still maintained a practice, though only three days a week. He was the entire medical staff of Rural Memorial Hospital, a 40-bed voluntary community facility that also was the major employer in Rural County. Attempts had been made by various community groups over the previous ten years to recruit additional physicians. On occasion, a foreign physician was attracted, but none were accepted by the community nor were they comfortable with the older physician, who dominated local hospital and medical affairs.

Virtually as a last resort, some community representatives approached University Hospital/Medical School (UHMS) and requested its assistance. By coincidence, officials at UHMS had been discussing the idea of rural primary care for some time. They recognized the pressing need for physicians in many rural areas of the state, and felt that if they could develop ways to meet that need, they would counter legislative concerns that they were not doing enough for their home state. Concerns had been expressed in the legislature over the number of out-of-state residents attending the medical school and the number of resident graduates leaving the state to practice.

As they envisioned it, a network of rural primary care centers could serve a number of useful functions:

- meeting rural health care needs
- upgrading quality of care in rural areas
- providing training sites for family practice residencies
- promoting support for UHMS as a significant community service
- assisting in budget discussions with the legislature
- enabling UHMS to demonstrate the value of its progressive approach to primary care
- attracting foundation and government grant funds to support UHMS programs

They believed the first center in such a network could be developed in Rural County. The faculty of the medical school, mainly the Department of Family Practice, had developed previously a design for a primary care center. It called for a staff of two or three physicians, augmented by a team of paraprofessionals: nurse practitioners and physician's assistants trained in the university's program. The design called for the paraprofessional to take some of the physicians' workload (taking histories, routine examinations, etc.) plus contributing their own unique services to patient education and health promotion.

Comprehensive family medical records would be developed, to include data on family health habits (smoking, drinking, diet, exercise), use of all health services (dental care, prescription and nonprescription drug use, psychiatric or other mental health services). The program would combine high quality and continuity of care for entire families and the community. It would demonstrate through its own records the effectiveness of the program in meeting rural health needs and would serve as the model for a network of similar centers throughout the state.

A BREAK WITH PAST PATTERNS

The design thus developed represented a sharp contrast from the previous patterns of medical care. The old-time practitioner tended to diagnose and treat each illness as it occurred, caring little for health education or prevention other than standard immunizations. Everyone who came, by appointment or walk-in, got to see the doctor eventually, though waits often were matters of hours. Individuals seen by the local physician always were given something for their problems: pills, shots, or prescriptions. They frequently were hospitalized for relatively minor conditions and kept in the hospital unusually long. In effect, the hospital served as a combination acute care and long-term care facility.

In contrast, the new program offered emphasis on ambulatory rather than inpatient care, on education and prevention rather than treatment. An appointment system was developed to prevent long waits, and educational messages were posted around the waiting room. Patients entering the center often would be seen by a physician's assistant and a nurse practitioner in addition to, and sometimes instead of, the physician. Administrative systems and procedures were designed to smooth patient flow, billing, recordkeeping, and management.

The program was begun slightly ahead of schedule when the local physician had a heart attack and had to give up his practice, leaving no one to serve the entire local population. A local church provided examining, treatment, and waiting room space at no charge to the center. While original plans called for a July 1 start-up, the center was able to open its doors and receive its first patient more than six months early. Despite opening in the slack Christmas period, the center was busy from its first day.

The center operated under the direction of a physician who had been recruited as a field professor of family practice on the faculty of UHMS. His salary was paid by the university, although receipts from the center offset this cost to a significant degree. Until full-time physicians became available, staffing was provided by the University Hospital residents on a rotating basis. Two physician's assistants and a nurse practitioner provided sufficient additional personnel to meet demands, although their time was allocated in the main to health promotion and education rather than diagnosis and treatment.

Weekend coverage and after-hours emergencies were handled by members of the faculty on an on-call basis, mostly via telephone. Home visits were made rarely, and only for absolutely bedridden patients, since travel time would cost, on average, ten times the time allocated per visit.

Within three months, the center was considered a success. Following only a few announcements of its opening in the county weekly newspaper and on local radio, patient volume had reached the break-even point in only three weeks. While paraprofessionals were busier giving care than intended because of the lack of full-time physicians, this situation would be remedied by July 1 when two physicians recruited for the center were to arrive. Income of the center was not covering its costs, but morale was high. When grant funds that had been sought through various government programs and foundations were approved, the future of the center and of a regional network of centers looked assured.

The local hospital, however, was not doing quite so well. With its new emphasis on prevention and ambulatory rather than inpatient care, the center was not referring half as many patients to Rural Memorial as previous physicians. Many patients were referred to UHMS, even for relatively routine care, in order to allow the center physicians to concentrate on the specific problems on which their training had focused. Length of stay for patients admitted to RMH was four days shorter, on average, than under the previous physician.

DECLINE IN OCCUPANCY, DELAY ON PAYMENTS

As a result, the hospital's occupancy dropped precipitously, from 64 percent in November to only 30 percent in April. The hospital board was forced to borrow money just to meet expenses. Payment of bills fell behind schedule and creditors complained. There were substantial staff layoffs, and supplies were pared to the bone. Despite the revenue generated for the hospital through its selling administrative and support services to the center, the financial situation became critical and the board members searched frantically for relief.

In an effort to assist the hospital, the university-sponsored primary care center began to allocate a portion of its budget for the hospital's administrative, support, and maintenance services. Members of the university's graduate program in hospital administration analyzed the RMH's financial difficulties and recommended that it convert to a nursing home. However, such a step was not acceptable to the hospital board, which felt that the community would not be served adequately since the nearest hospital was 37 miles away over poor roads.

When the two young physicians recruited to be full-time staff at the primary care center visited Rural County in May, they received sharply contrasting impressions. The center was busy and staff morale seemed high. However, patients complained, often bitterly, about being talked to instead of treated. They recalled nostalgically how things had been with the old physician and couldn't understand or accept the new style of program at the center. The hospital was in desperate straits, and the board of trustees in a panic.

One of the conditions imposed by the grant that supported the program was that physicians would have to be salaried, with a maximum starting salary of $40,000 a year. When apprised of this fact, the two young physicians became angry. Original discussions had suggested both a higher starting salary and a sharing by the physicians of any surplus revenues generated by high volume. Despite the fact that the center was losing money at the time, the two physicians felt it could become a very successful practice with some changes in staffing.

When the university proved unable or unwilling to compromise on compensation, the two physicians refused to sign a contract and instead decided to set up practice on their own. Within days of opening their office, they were busy, and soon their admissions to the hospital increased occupancy significantly. As patient volume disappeared, the center's prospects died and the university's interest in and support for it dwindled. A review by the UHMS administration concluded that local health needs were being met adequately by the two new private practitioners and decided that the center should close. By September, the center no longer existed, having operated for only a little more than eight months.

ANALYSIS

From a marketing perspective, UHMS's approach to primary care program development did almost everything wrong, yet almost succeeded. The flaws in this approach will be described in terms of the four major components of program design in a marketing construct: product, place, price, and promotion.

Product

A marketing approach requires that the market or community be examined first in an effort to identify what they are most interested in buying or using. In contrast, UHMS designed well in advance, and independent of the realities of Rural County, a primary care program *it* wanted to develop. It had its product first and was just looking for a market to sell it to. This was a *sales* orientation rather than a marketing one. It did not attempt to identify what the community wanted and then provide an appropriate design, but determined paternalistically what the community *should* want and decided to offer it.

The product actually developed missed being what the community wanted in a number of ways. In contrast to the hands-on, mysterious science of diagnosis and treatment, the primary care center offered education and insisted individuals change their habits. In contrast to extended rest in the local hospital from the stresses of crowded and underheated homes, the center offered ambulatory care and sent the patients back to the grind immediately or referred them to the distant University Hospital. Instead of a single father figure familiar with each family member, the primary care center offered a touring company of different rotating specialists and teams of paraprofessionals who had to look up everybody's name in the records.

From the hospital's perspective, instead of a loyal medical staff that kept the beds filled, the center staff referred only occasional short stays and sent many patients off to the University Hospital. Instead of stable occupancy and income, the center brought financial disaster. Where the previous physician had provided stable jobs and income for hospital employees and pharmacists, the center offered them a local depression.

Place

The location of the primary care center was, if anything, ideal. It was next to the hospital facility and convenient to travel patterns and the hospital's laboratory and x-ray services. However, home visits were eliminated, even though many nonbedridden patients had enjoyed them in the past. The appointment system failed to accommodate the casual local attitude about time and discouraged walk-ins. Under the new system, individuals had to wait twice—for an appointment, then, upon arriving at the center, to be seen. The hours of operation reflected the times the center employees preferred to work, not when local residents wanted to call.

Price

The price to local residents for primary care center services represented a significant departure from the past. Charges for ambulatory services were lower than for inpatient care, but Medicare, Medicaid, and health insurance failed to cover many outpatient services completely, so the out-of-pocket cost to each consumer actually increased. Moreover, patients were given care often apparently unrelated to their immediate complaint, and the feeling was widespread that local citizens were being used as guinea pigs in some research project.

Promotion (Communication)

Promotional efforts by the center were minimal in the conventional sense: radio and newspaper advertising. Certainly no attempt was made to promote two-way communication to aid in program design or monitoring. The ad hoc community group that originally had approached UHMC for help was not used as a permanent advisory or feedback mechanism. No effort was expended at explaining the nature and benefits of the primary care center's new approach to medical care delivery. The community was expected to recognize and welcome the superiority of the university's methods as self-evidently worthwhile.

COMPETITION: THE COUP DE GRACE

What really did the center in, of course, was competition. In the short run, because of the virtually complete absence of competition, the primary care center was busy and, in its own eyes, successful. It was only when the two new physicians developed an effective competitive offering that the center's failings became critical.

It often is true, in health care as in other industries, that the only product available sells well until a better alternative comes along. Being first in time to reach the market normally is a tremendous advantage, but only where you come close to offering product/price benefits roughly equal to those who come later. Once everyone in the area had tried the center's program, they knew what its product was, and it was so unsatisfactory as to drive patients to the first alternative that came along. Had no alternative developed, the center might be there still.

DISCUSSION

The failure of the center to meet its market's expectations went well beyond its providing primary care services to patients. By failing to supply sufficient inpatients, it threatened the hospital and, with it, the largest employer in the county. Employees lost their jobs in an already depressed area and hospital employee morale plummeted. The hospital board, made up of powerful local leaders, felt betrayed by those it had turned to for help. It was clear to the community at large that the university was doing its own thing, not seeing to the best interests of the local residents.

The issue of pandering to misplaced perceptions vs. doing what's best for people is raised clearly by this case. It probably could be argued very effectively that the university's approach was far superior technically to that of the two new physicians in terms of the community's best health interests. Where unnecessary admissions and overly long stays existed, the community was paying a premium for having its hospital, though so indirectly it might not be aware of it. The educational services and promotional efforts of the center might have been far better for patients than ritualistic vitamin shots, placebos, or dubious prescriptions.

The health care provider has a unique dilemma relative to marketing. Do you deliver what's best or what will sell? Other industries rarely face this problem. Unless a product that will sell is clearly illegal (heroin, marijuana, prostitution, etc.) or strongly objectionable morally (sugar cereals for children, alcohol, tobacco) marketing what will sell is not criticized even mildly. For health care, however, providers have a professional responsibility to do what's best for the patient, not pander to uninformed whims.

If all choices were of a dilemma nature, between doing what's right even if it doesn't sell or doing what's wrong because it does, health care would be in a terrible fix. Fortunately, most choices lie between these two extremes. There are ways we can modify programs to meet expectations, and can influence expectations to be closer to what is "best for people."

In this case, the health care needs of the community should have been treated more comprehensively. Rather than considering primary care as a single, isolated program, it should have been viewed as part of the entire health and economic system. The full impact of its approach on the hospital and the financial as well as the physical health of the community should have been considered. Rather than contriving to fill the hospital via dubious admissions or overextended stays, the facility might have been kept occupied by converting some beds to long-term care. In a community with large numbers of aged, the need for nursing home care is likely to be substantial.

It might not have been necessary to adopt 50-year-old medicine in order to meet patient expectations. Two temporary full-time physicians rather than a rotating troupe could have filled the interim period before two permanent physicians arrived. These physicians could have weaned the patients gradually away from the "always-treat-em" patterns of the past rather than insisting on a radical new approach right off the bat. If steps had been designed gradually, with effective communication to and from community residents and hospital board members, change might very well have been introduced without destroying either the center or the hospital.

Only by recognizing the complete agendas of communities served, medical and social, psychological as well as physical, economic as well as health, are new programs or substantial changes likely to succeed. It is very difficult for outside agencies such as UHMS and its faculty to identify and appreciate the full range of perceived needs among a community. Had the university adopted a more listening than lecturing attitude toward the community, it might have learned enough to avoid serious errors. Employment of a community advisory board to act as codesigner rather than supplicant might have enlisted greater support and improved program design.

The only sensible approach to dealing with conflicts between what is good for people and what will sell is compromise. Unless professionals are so persuasive as to convert consumers by promotional efforts alone, health care products, prices, and places will have to be modified to meet local expectations as well as professional standards. Such compromises are most likely to occur and be accepted when they take place in a setting where providers and consumers play roles as codesigners of new programs, where each accepts its right and obligation to educate and be educated by the other.

MARKETING: THE CRITICAL FACTOR

The most critical problems related to primary care development often are immersed in hospital relations. Primary care programs sponsored by hospitals have made significant inroads in rural and even in underserved urban areas, but not without some bruises to show for it. Plans by a hospital to develop a program may be supported strongly when an obvious shortage of primary care physicians exists, then support may dry up if the shortage diminishes through private recruiting, National Health Service Corps, etc., or if the local economy takes a downturn.

Hospital medical staff members most likely to welcome primary care developments are the specialists, provided they are confident referrals from primary care centers will be distributed equitably. Less likely to support such programs are other primary practitioners (general or family practitioners, pediatricians, and obstetricians) who may view the centers as competition. Where staff for the centers must be recruited through financial guarantees, special perquisites, etc., the medical staff may feel much like veteran athletes seeing the rookies get enormous salaries.

The potential rewards to the hospital of primary care programs should not be oversold. Many such centers fail to break even, though they may be justified if their resulting increased referrals produce sufficient marginal revenue to make up the difference. Third party organizations are becoming increasingly wary of accepting losses from primary care programs in reimbursable costs, or are insisting upon counting net income from such programs as an offset to inpatient costs.

In many areas, the success of a center promotes problems. When patient volume and revenue become great, the physicians employed in the center may decide to strike out on their own. Patients are likely to feel closer to the physicians than to the center, and follow them to their new locations, leaving the center empty. In the case described, the center's success under a temporary arrangement demonstrated to the two recruits that a sufficient population and income potential existed for private practice, but in a different mode.

Intelligent marketing should be directed at deciding whether a primary care program is a desirable, feasible, and optimal idea, as well as at developing the most promising approach to its development. Since primary care, more than any other level of health service, requires the active cooperation of consumers, marketing is even more critical to its success than for other health service programs.

Chapter 18

An Urban Primary Care Center

Both urban and rural areas have seen the development of hospital-sponsored primary care programs in response to severe shortages of private physicians. While underserved urban areas have certain advantages over rural (higher population density, better transportation), they also have disadvantages (low income, cultural heterogeneity). The marketing challenge is the same, however: identifying and responding to the product, price, and place in which the market is most interested, thereby effectively meeting community needs.

The case of Urban Medical Center (UMC) is a composite of the author's experiences with a number of urban primary care programs. It is intended to convey a number of typical developmental problems and opportunities and to suggest marketing responses that may prove worth considering. While it focuses on a hospital's development of a primary care satellite, the principles and lessons contained should be equally applicable to any organization considering such a development.

A CHANGING COMMUNITY

Urban Medical Center is a 320-bed acute care general hospital with a history of more than 100 years' service to the community. It has grown over the years from a source of general acute care for the immediate surroundings to a regional medical center emphasizing specialty services such as cardiovascular surgery and physical medicine and rehabilitation, and treating patients from a four-state area. It still retains a strong community mission, however, and more than 80 percent of its admissions are residents of the metropolitan area.

Like many downtown hospitals, UMC has seen recent changes in its own neighborhood. Once a fashionable residential area, the neighborhood with the passage of time has shifted toward increasingly lower socioeconomic groups. As a result, it now contains a mix of residents: older hangovers from middle class whites, more recently arrived blacks, and the even more recently arrived Hispanics, Indians, and Asians. The level of transiency is high, as are unemployment and illiteracy.

UMC is the southernmost hospital in the downtown area, though only by a matter of blocks. As urban sprawl has spread to the south, it became the logical choice for the entire south side, as no hospital exists in that part of the city. However, medical staff members at UMC practice in more fashionable areas, in the main, so relatively few of their inpatients come from the south side. However, more than 50 percent of their emergency room visitors are residents of the immediate area.

The two major competitors for UMC are Doctors Hospital and Memorial Medical Clinic and Hospital (MMCH). Doctors concentrates primarily on surgery and has built up a strong referral network through its residency training programs. MMCH has its own multispecialty group practice of 120 physicians and a network arrangement with a large number of rural hospitals to promote and facilitate referrals. UMC is a rather typical independent institution, relying on its attending staff to bring in an adequate number of admissions.

Gradually, it became clear to UMC that if it wished to maintain a strong referral/specialist function in the community, it must beef up its primary care referral base. As a first step, it developed a family practice residency training program as the local medical school expanded its program and avidly sought additional residency sites. It also shifted from rotating staff to contract coverage of its emergency room. This both relieved the medical staff of onerous duty and set the precedent for hospital employment of primary care physicians.

The next logical step was to develop its own primary care program. The first choice, in most cases, would have been to develop an onsite primary care program to handle the routine cases in the emergency room. Two factors mitigated against this choice, however. First, a relatively small proportion of the visits was truly routine, only 30 to 40 percent in contrast to the 60 to 70 percent typical of urban hospital emergency rooms. Second, the medical staff general and family practitioners were reluctant to sponsor an onsite competitor.

The next obvious choice was to locate sources of primary care in the south side. Three sites looked promising. With a population of 90,000 and only 15 full-time physicians, all generalists, the south side probably could support another dozen or so physicians. The hospital could sponsor three primary care programs of 3 to 4 physicians each and anticipate adequate utilization of all of them. Using the government standard of one physician per 3,500 population as a bare minimum, the area should support 26 physicians. Using the commonly accepted optimum of one physician per 1,500 individuals, as many as 60 could be justified.

The prospect of gambling on three separate primary care programs, however, seemed to frighten the board of trustees and greatly distress the medical staff, especially the specialists. They saw such a development to be a major shift from traditional emphasis on specialty care and feared that too much capital and attention would be drawn away from the more important specialty service programs. Similarly, while the board generally was supportive of the idea, members were reluctant to take as big a gamble as opening three centers without some thorough study.

ENTER THE CONSULTANT

A consultant was employed to do a more careful analysis of market prospects for primary care, including a financial feasibility study for a specific program. In addition, representatives of community organizations in the south side were approached to enlist their aid and support in developing the program.

The initial response of residents of the community was skeptical and somewhat suspicious. They perceived the hospital as primarily a "carriage trade" institution lacking any demonstrated commitment to serving the residents of the south side. Moreover, each of the different ethnic groups in the community had its own notion as to what kind of program should be developed and who should run it.

In addition to the 15 private physicians serving the south side, there were a number of public clinics. The city health department sponsored a clinic that provided specific categorical services, primarily to the black population: maternal and child care, children and youth services, family planning, etc. This represented a free but fragmented source of primary care, serving primarily women and young children.

There also existed a program offering services to the Indian members of the community, sponsored by the U.S. Indian Health Service. A "free clinic" had been organized to serve the Spanish-speaking residents, although its hours of operation were infrequent and unpredictable. None of these programs offered services at any but normal working hours, five days a week. Each had its own idea, however, about the major needs and best sites for any new program, and resented UMC's rather late demonstration of interest.

The lack of support by community groups represented a real barrier in two different ways. First, the lack of such support could result in negative action by the local Health Systems Agency to any certificate of need required in developing the primary care program. Second, animosity among the community organizations might well result in low use of any program actually developed.

UMC decided to combine its two major concerns (market analysis and community support) by sponsoring a communitywide study of primary care needs. The hospital offered the use of its consultant, planning staff, and computer to the community organizations so that both could get a fuller picture of local needs. Each organization contributed suggestions for information to be collected, while the design of questionnaires, survey techniques, sampling, etc., was put in the hands of the consultant. The local university was invited to participate, and contributed advice and students to conduct interviews in the community.

This jointly sponsored survey produced some interesting results. Some of the services that the hospital considered to be of high priority interest (family planning, for one) were found to be low in the eyes of the community.

The chief barriers to care identified in the survey were cultural and financial. Nonwhite residents of the area encountered both language and acceptance difficulties when seeking care among the local private physicians, all of whom were white. Many of these physicians were accepting no additional Medicaid patients, although few actually were overworked. Indians and Asians in the community did not like going to the public health clinic, which they saw as a black-oriented program. Even for the free clinics, the cost of transportation, lost time from work, or difficulty finding babysitters proved financial barriers.

Following up the survey, UMC invited the community organizations to send representatives to serve on a community advisory board for the primary care program. This was designed to firm up community support and ensure that the program stayed in tune with community needs. It proved to be a source of problems as well.

First off, the community organizations were used to serving on governing boards for the neighborhood health centers and free clinics. They were not satisfied initially with a purely advisory role and tended to try to make policy and operational decisions. Moreover, they clearly had agendas that went beyond developing a primary care program. They put pressure on the hospital to hire no one but community residents to work in the program and to include welfare and legal advice to residents along with health care. Each of the minority groups insisted that physicians employed in the program be from its minority.

Private physicians in the area also put up some resistance. While all recognized the general shortage of primary care physicians in the area, none wanted the hospital to locate a center anywhere near their own practices. None of the free clinics wanted the hospital's competition too near, either. Each of the alternative sites being discussed tended to be disfavored by at least a number of significant individuals or groups.

STRATEGY

As administration at UMC realized the complexity and multiple potential pitfalls in developing the primary care program, it decided that it was too important to be relegated to marginal, part-time attention. Once it felt that the board was committed, the medical staff and community receptive in principle, and the idea basically sound, it hired a medical director to oversee the detailed development. This involved a significant gamble but administration felt there were a number of advantages to having a director early:

- A physician would be able to work more easily with the UMC medical staff and other providers in the community.

- The hiring of a physician would demonstrate a firm commitment to primary care without representing a substantial or irrevocable investment.

- A full-time director could devote the attention necessary to touch bases with all important publics.

- There were, however, some drawbacks to the idea in practice:

- The physician actually hired tended to be aggressive and somewhat abrasive, though energetic and highly motivated.

- The physician started with a pretty firm notion of what the primary program should be; substantial administrative and community pressures were needed to introduce some flexibility and situation-specific responsiveness into program design.

The community advisory board proved helpful in this. While members often disagreed among themselves, they refused to permit the medical director to dictate how the program should be developed. By insisting that this board approve major program decisions and site selection, the hospital ensured that basic market analysis and strategic thinking would be done.

While south side residents gradually came to give at least lukewarm support to the program, the metropolitan planning council did not. Fearing a negative action on any certificate-of-need application, and not wanting to build in substantial delay, UMC arranged to carry out the program development so that no certificate approval was necessary. By leasing rather than purchasing space, and locating the program under the family practice residency service, the hospital avoided having to get any external approvals. This strategy had its negative repercussions later, however. The HSA tended to view any subsequent certificate-of-need application from UMC with disfavor, making it doubly difficult to get approvals on other capital expenditures.

As it became obvious that local private physicians could have significant impact on the success of the program, the medical director found ways to capture the support of at least two. One physician was recruited to become a member of the staff of the center, with the promise that members of his office staff also would become employees of the center if they wished. Another physician, ready to retire, was encouraged to refer his former patients to the center when the medical director agreed to lease the office owned by the physician as the center's first location. It was recognized that subsequent expansion might require additional quarters, but the retiring physician was happy to see that his former patients could receive care in an accustomed place.

The program of the primary care center was geared to the needs of the immediate population and to the market positions left open by competing providers. In addition to basic primary care, the center offers the services of an obstetrician and a pediatrician who hold scheduled office hours there every week. The center's hours are 1 p.m. through 9 p.m. daily, and 8 a.m. till noon on Saturday, favoring the low income employed residents of the community.

The center also offers a 24-hour telephone response service, with referral to the UMC emergency room if immediate attention is warranted. A special van makes scheduled stops throughout the area on an hourly basis, picking up and returning patients who lack their own cars or are far from public transport.

In addition to the white physician recruited from among the available providers, two minority physicians were hired, one black and one Hispanic. Local residents were recruited actively for center jobs, and four are employed there, although the staff does not consist exclusively of local residents. The staff is quite representative of the racial mix of the local population, however.

The four physicians were hired initially on a salaried basis. Suspecting that this arrangement would be accepted on only a short-term basis, however, UMC developed an incentive contract arrangement that was put into effect during the third year of operation. By that time, volume had reached the point where it might have appeared attractive for one or more of the physicians to strike out individually. The incentive contract, worked out in conjunction with the physicians themselves, prevented such defection.

The medical director left, however, to develop a similar program in another area. This was not felt to be a negative occurrence. His interests, personality, and talents lay chiefly in development, not in day-to-day management. His aggressive, often abrasive style was useful in making sure things got done but was beginning to cause problems with the board and medical staff. Many of the routine administrative functions were taken over by the hospital. The new medical director was expected to spend most of his time in delivering care rather than in administration.

The center refers patients requiring specialist services to one of the specialists on UMC's medical staff. The prospect of additional referrals was the factor that turned around the opposition of the specialists. Instead of viewing the primary care center as an unwarranted displacement of emphasis on generalist services, they came to see it as a major source of new business. By concentrating the program in an underserved area, fears of the hospital's generalists that the center would be unwelcome competition were defused. Moreover, the center provides reports on after-hours emergency calls and emergency room visits to the local practitioners when one of their patients is treated.

The hospital perceives two distinct benefits arising from the center. First, it is bringing in new business to the hospital: referrals for laboratory and x-ray services (though all routine lab and x-ray work is done at the center) plus referrals for the specialist medical staff and inpatient care. Second, the identification of the medical staff with and dependence on the hospital have been increased significantly. Including the family practice residency program and emergency room staff, there are 16 full-time primary care physicians under contract to the hospital. These generate many referrals to specialists and also bring in their own patients. Thus, gradually, the hospital is strengthening its hold on its sources of patients.

Financially, the center is not yet an unqualified success. Because of the low income levels and poor health insurance coverage of most of the south side residents, collections are slow and bad debt write-offs high. While volume is adequate, it is not sufficient to produce revenue equal to expenses.

To some extent, the hospital is gambling on the future. When a comprehensive national health insurance program is implemented, revenues are expected to at least meet expenditures. With the referrals generated to the hospital for inpatient care, break-even operation of the center would be considered a significant success. Moreover, by developing the first hospital-sponsored primary care program in the area, UMC stands to have a head start when national health insurance makes the area attractive to competitors.

The center is proving a source of pride to the board of trustees and a helpful advantage in recruiting medical staff and attracting family practice residents. Each of the residents is given an opportunity to rotate through the center to experience practice away from the hospital. Specialists are attracted more easily when they see UMC's strong commitment to ensuring a supply of referrals.

DISCUSSION

UMC has used a combination of deliberate and unconscious marketing approaches in developing its primary care center. Basically, it has followed a philosophy of finding out what the market wants and trying to respond accordingly:

- Medical staff members were given referrals (specialists) or feedback on care of their patients (generalists) in return for their support or at least tacit approval of the program.
- Community organizations were given jobs and services aimed at the expressed wishes of their constituencies in return for their support.
- The board of trustees was given a source of pride and a financially positive, though not self-supporting, program in return for its support.
- Administration increased its power and improved the financial prospects of the hospital in return for its hard work.
- Community residents were given an additional source of care and such new products as evening hours, 24-hour phone service, and obstetric and pediatric care in return for their patronage.
- Local physicians were given jobs, after-hours coverage, and a cooperating colleague rather than a competitor in return for their support.
- The HSA, while originally an enemy of the program, was swayed by the measurable improvement in health status and by the community acceptance of the program.

DISCUSSION QUESTIONS

1. In developing a primary care program, whose behavior is success dependent upon:
   a. community groups?
   b. potential patients?
   c. local physicians?
   d. planning/regulatory agencies?
   e. insurance/government programs?
   f. professionals to be recruited?
   g. others?
2. What incentives or exchanges will the program by its very nature offer to any of these groups in return for their favorable action?
3. What incentives or exchanges can you design into the program or your strategy for its development so as to win the favorable action you require?
4. What are the costs/benefits of providing such incentives?
5. How serious would be a failure to achieve favorable action from any one group?

Chapter 19

A Guide to Developing Primary Care Programs

The author's experience in the use of marketing concepts and techniques has been concentrated in the area of hospital-sponsored primary care programs. Based on such experience, this discussion attempts to identify factors to be considered and specific marketing strategies that might be employed in developing primary care programs. While this discussion is oriented toward hospital sponsorship of primary medical care programs, it should provide helpful insights for anyone developing programs that serve the public directly.

The conceptual approach used in addressing the development of primary care programs contains the following steps:

1. Decide what constitutes success for a primary care program—specific parameters and indicators that will inform you whether the program is working, should be maintained or expanded, or should be discontinued

2. Identify the key actions, events, and circumstances that will determine whether or not the program becomes a success.

3. Identify preexisting situations or strategies you might employ that will make critical actions, events, and circumstances more or less probable.

4. Analyze alternative opportunities and select appropriate strategies that will produce the program most likely to be successful.

This model is a version of a common planning technique: specifying the desired future, then identifying the causal events and relationships that will produce that future. This backward-from-the-outcome thinking then becomes forward-from-the-present action so as to achieve the desired result. The marketing contribution to this approach comes from its focus on behavior and understanding of motivation in terms of exchange relationships.

1. IDENTIFYING SUCCESS PARAMETERS

While each organization should and typically does determine its own measures of success, some common indicators will be used here for the sake of illustration. Generally speaking, such measures reflect the health of the community or population served and the health of the institution itself. Depending on the type of program, health status measures related to preventable disease incidence, infant and material mortality, life expectancy and death rates, disability or self-perceived health may be employed. Measures reflecting the status of the entire population or specific market segments may be used.

The health of the organization is likely to be reflected in terms of traditional financial measures and market activity. These may include total revenue and expense, costs per units of specific services, accounts receivable, bad debts, net income, and changes over time, as well as total number of visits, registrants or active patients, new patients, missed appointments, service use per visit, etc.

In addition to financial and utilization measures, criteria reflecting quality and acceptability are likely to be considered. Process quality measures such as the number of patient records peer-reviewed each month may be employed. The results of peer reviews then may provide outcome measures of quality. Satisfaction levels as reflected in both subjective ratings by patients and objective behavior (repeat visits, compliance with prescribed behavior) can be used as measures of acceptability.

The more precisely and thoroughly such criteria for success are identified, the better. Ideally, standards also should be set for each criterion, but this is a much more complex process. The criteria often will be found to conflict with each other—higher quality requiring greater costs, higher acceptability raising expenditures, faster growth reducing quality, etc. It is more important that appropriate and useful criteria be identified and employed than rigid standards be imposed. Most frequently, standards are compromised in practice when the extent of conflict among criteria or constraints of the real world are felt.

For example, a hospital-sponsored primary care program may have its success defined in terms of being profitable or self-supporting as a specific institutional program. However, it may be found that when the hospital's overhead costs are apportioned, the program fails to achieve such a status. Success then may be redefined as achieving break-even status for direct costs, especially if indirect costs can be reapportioned among cost-based reimbursement departments. Even if the program fails to break even on its direct costs, it may be termed a success if it generates sufficient referrals for inpatient and ancillary services to create a net financial benefit, or at least no net financial harm, to the hospital.

Ultimately, the test of success comes in determining whether or not the institution and its community would be better off with or without the program. When this test is applied, it may turn out that a program that is a financial failure by any standard still should be maintained for its net benefit to the community and hospital. As costs and reimbursement are regulated increasingly, the support of financially negative programs will become increasingly difficult. As long as any chance of private philanthropy or community support exists, however, such programs are potentially viable. It may well become common for local communities to dig into their own pockets to support programs that government-dictated reimbursement fails to finance adequately. Such support becomes the ultimate test of market success.

2. IDENTIFYING KEY CONDITIONS

Once the nature of success has been determined, it should be possible to identify fairly precisely the set of conditions that will produce that success (possible, though not necessarily easy). For example, to produce a given financial outcome, some combination of revenue and expense is required. To achieve a target level of expenditures, some specific amounts for facilities, personnel, equipment, and supplies must not be exceeded. To achieve a target revenue level, some specific number of visits and revenue per visit must occur. To generate some revenue per visit, some specific charge per visit and collection relationship must be established.

The process of identifying such conditions is, in effect, the generation of a causal construct, describing how certain behaviors (your productivity, their utilization) leads to certain outcomes. In theory, there are literally infinite possible interlocking conditions that might produce the same successful outcome. For example, there are countless combinations of revenue and expense that will produce the same net profit, countless combinations of visits and income per visit that will produce the same revenue.

In practice, however, the number of possibilities that realistically must be examined is limited easily. Revenue per visit is likely to be comparable to existing programs, the number of visits limited by the target population, and so on. Many of the items in the complex of relationships that produce success will be fixed early or are related closely. The size of the facility is limited to the number of staff members employed, and the charge per visit is constrained by the competition, reimbursement policies, and expected impact on demand.

Typically, the most important determinants of success will emerge from this analysis and become the focus of further investigation. For a primary care program, such determinants are likely to include:

- obtaining a facility whose cost, amenities, and location are optimal
- recruiting professionals who can provide some quality and quantity of production
- attracting sufficient customers and utilization to match the facility and professionals in terms of productivity and revenue vs. expense
- obtaining the necessary support and approvals from critical groups: hospital medical staff, board of trustees, local government, planning, and reimbursement authorities

Each of these is related closely. Where a facility is found will influence how many individuals will come, based on distance. How many come will influence how many professionals are required. How many professionals are employed will influence what facility is required. The combination of facility and professional costs vs. customer revenue will influence the support received and approval necessary.

A marketing approach tends to begin with customers, where a conventional planning approach might begin with a program design. How many customers are there, potentially? Where do they live and what do they do now with regard to use of proposed services? What amount of service utilization might be expected under optimum conditions?

3. IDENTIFYING CONTRIBUTING CONDITIONS

Once critical behaviors have been delineated, factors that would tend to facilitate vs. hinder such behaviors should be identified. The extent to which such factors are present or absent, or can be introduced as a market strategy by the organization, will then be analyzed. In effect, this step asks whether the sets of behavior that will produce a successful program are inherently likely and/or can be promoted by actions that the organization can take.

Attracting Customers

The probability of attracting customers is always the most critical concern in employing a marketing approach. The factors that affect consumer behavior and the current state of such factors in the available markets must be examined first. Where a specific market is being analyzed preparatory to a go/no-go decision on a specific program, the status of critical causal factors should determine whether success is probable enough to warrant going ahead. Where a number of markets is being analyzed, the optimal alternative(s) can be identified in terms of their probability of successfully attracting customers.

The key to primary care development is to recognize that patients are customers. They are the people who decide whether to use a specific service: where, when, how, and from whom. It is the nature of their motivation and the probability of their behavior that indicates whether a given program will succeed.

The second key reality that must be addressed is the fact that wherever individuals perceive a need, they should be presumed to be coping with that need somehow. In other words, even if your program proposes a service not now available within 50 miles of the population you're examining, you still should recognize that you've got competition. People are either traveling that 50 miles to the current source, or they're substituting other services: the local druggist, retired nurse, chiropractor, or faith healer as sources of medical care.

It is essential, therefore, that you discover first whether or not customers perceive the need for the service you propose. If not, you may have a big job of education/motivation to do in generating any demand at all for your program. If so, you've got to offer individuals something they will perceive as better than their current arrangement: superior product, price, or place.

This means that basic research must be done to ascertain the current behaviors and attitudes of your target market. What you'd like to discover through such research is information on such factors as whether there is:

- a chiefly younger, highly mobile population—less likely to have strong attachments to other programs
- good insurance coverage or income
- a relatively well-educated population with high awareness of the value of the service you propose
- high dissatisfaction with the current source of services because of access or the cost of quality factors that you can provide better
- interest in establishing a regular source of service, rather than merely a local stopgap or episodic source

Research also should extend to the nature, current developments, and future plans of existing and potential competitors. What you'd like to find is whether:

- local sources of similar services are seriously overtaxed, plan to retire, or can be enticed to become part of your program, bringing their patients with them

- potential competitors are lacking interest, have a history of not being able to move quickly, have a poor reputation locally, don't have resources to develop a competing program, etc.

Recruiting Professionals

Assuming all or a sufficient number of market factors are positive, the ability to provide the services potentially in demand is dependent on recruiting the appropriate quantity and quality of professionals. The professionals you'd want are likely to be:

- interested in living where your market is, so as to achieve social links with prospective patients
- younger, and interested in staying in the area
- positive in attitude toward the kind of organizational arrangement you can offer rather than likely to strike off on their own
- willing to participate or take the lead in attracting patients rather than expecting you to bring them all in

In addition to factors that make the market look positive to you, the elements that might make it positive or negative to professionals also should be examined. What are the local schools, recreational resources, social amenities like? What kinds of housing are available? What arrangements can be made for coverage during the day, weekends, holidays, and vacations? What opportunities exist or can be arranged for interactions with peers?

You can influence greatly the attraction that the opportunity your program represents holds for professionals. Salaried arrangements are likely to be much less attractive than contracts that provide a guaranteed minimum income plus strong incentives for building patient volume. Greater independence is likely to be more attractive than programs tightly integrated into a larger, centralized organization, and flexible, negotiated approaches more attractive than standardized policies and procedures.

In general, you should focus on what you have to offer and how it might be made superior to other alternatives the professionals you want to recruit might have. In an organized program, you can offer established facilities, equipment, an attractive market, guaranteed (but not limited) income, limited responsibility, evening/weekend/vacation coverage, or whatever attracts professionals to organized systems rather than to private practice.

An optimal arrangement might be to recruit a local practitioner who can become a full-time member of the program staff or perhaps spend the last six months or a year before retirement in your program, gradually turning over patients until retirement comes. Such an approach is likely to guarantee a large patient volume immediately, rather than the slower alternative of starting from scratch. Of course, it may compromise the program you have in mind since both the local practitioner and patients are used to current practice. The costs vs. benefits of such a strategy should be evaluated carefully.

Acquiring Facilities

The location, layout, amenities, and cost of facilities are critical factors in program development. Because most programs start slowly, burdening them with a very expensive facility at the outset may make it difficult to achieve financial success. At the same time, an unattractive or inadequate facility may create problems in attracting patients at the outset or cause expansion difficulties later. Usually, it is more dangerous to be too big than too small, however. Foundation or bequest support that encourages organizations to build expensive, large, and overequipped facilities often does a disservice. While a program can expand gradually via construction or relocation, it is hard (if not impossible) to contract.

An optimal opportunity might be to take over the office and practice of an existing physician upon retirement or together with the practitioner. Even if the space might be less than perfect, the familiar location and linkage to an established practice may be an advantage.

Failing this, a location in or near a nexus of travel patterns is desirable. A shopping center may be particularly attractive, especially if its developer chose the site based on effective analysis of travel patterns. Adequate parking is a positive factor, as is any location that people routinely pass. The constant cue of a convenient location will remind residents of your existence and promote remembrance of appointments.

In many communities, public support for primary care programs may be evidenced by willingness to offer existing space or even to build a facility at no cost to you. Such a gesture not only offers a distinct cost advantage but also carries with it the likelihood of strong support and interest by local influentials. The offer should be examined, however, to be sure such advantages are not overshadowed by considerations of location, layout, size, etc.

Gaining Support and Approval

The number of publics whose support and approval are likely to be necessary to a successful primary care program is increasing continually. For a hospital, the board and medical staff as well as administration can make or break a program at the outset. The potential costs and benefits to each of such a program, and opportunities to modify them in program design, should be weighed carefully.

The hospital board may be won over by potential financial consequences, the opportunity for growth, the chance to expand service to the community. The role of the hospital as well as the interests of each of the board members should be examined in terms of how they would or could be affected, preferably furthered, by the proposed program. Giving some members a role in development, naming the program after a respected citizen, or other direct exchanges of values are possible.

The medical staff may well be opposed to or mildly disinterested in such a program. Primary practitioners on the staff may see the program as direct competition or object to the special treatment offered physicians recruited for the programs. Locating the program far from their practices or offering each the opportunity to serve in the program may dull opposition. Arranging to have program physicians cover for staff members, or referring them patients on occasion, also may help.

Specialists might object on one of two grounds: either because the hospital is using resources for primary care that could be devoted to specialized programs, or out of concern over who will get referrals from the primary care program. The number of potential referrals, if sufficient, should reduce their opposition in general, although special arrangements may have to be made to ensure that referrals are made in a way they consider equitable. The support of the medical staff may not always be achieved at the outset. If not, the hospital should at least be sure that the effect of the program eventually will be seen as, on the whole, positive.

Approval of the community in which the program is proposed is a separate matter. Local zoning variance or other formal approval is likely to be required in addition to community interest as a basis for generating sufficient utilization. Naming the program after the community or an honored resident may help. Setting up a local community advisory board to participate in planning the program also is likely to prove helpful. (The same comment applies to the board and medical staff—their participation in planning the program should smooth their eventual acceptance and support.)

Regulatory and planning agencies may have to be included. Approvals for reimbursement by government and private insurance programs should be investigated and pursued early. Certificate-of-need or other regulatory approvals should be considered even earlier. Published plans and policies of such organizations should provide clues as to the criteria they will use. In general, primary care programs that can be shown to promise reductions in total health care costs are likely to be shoo-ins. Programs that promise only improvements in access and/or quality are less certain. The existence and demonstration of strong support by the community to be served is likely to be very influential in regulatory decisions.

Funding for development or subsidization of such programs should be sought carefully. While the prospect of hundreds of thousands of dollars in "free" grants may seem overpoweringly attractive, they are likely to be a mixed blessing. First off, there's bound to be a tendency to spend someone else's money more freely and carelessly than your own. This may promote overdevelopment in facilities, equipment, or personnel that impose difficult burdens on long-range operation of the program. Second, the grants are likely to contain significant constraints that may be at variance with your own philosophy or that may interfere with the ultimate success of the program.

Requirements that physicians be paid salaries may make it difficult to attract physicians or may promote their leaving the organization and going into business for themselves as soon as utilization builds. External emphasis on underserved populations may make it difficult to attract sufficient paying patients. Government involvement, by itself, may raise the hackles of the local community or medical staff, on top of whatever conditions it imposes.

In general, all gifts should be examined for overall cost benefit. Each compromise with what an optimal program would be like, made in the interests of receiving immediate support, may reduce seriously the long-range viability of the program. Obviously, support that focuses on outcomes and is geared to helping you design a program suited to local realities is superior to support that focuses on process and dictates a standardized approach regardless of local circumstances.

The value of such support in expanding your vision and spurring your efforts should not be ignored, however. Some grants will force you to look at the opportunity more broadly, perhaps expanding the services provided or population served to the greater benefit of all. Others, by promoting a "jump in with both feet" rather than a "toe in the water" approach may push you to greater effort and ultimately to success beyond what you thought possible. There always is the danger, however, that external support will push you too far or in the wrong direction, so gift horses should be looked in the mouth.

4. STRATEGIC CHOICES AND DEVELOPMENT

By examining each opportunity in terms of the preexistence or potential promotion of conditions that enhance the probability of success, you can decide whether or which opportunity should be pursued. Moreover, analysis of such conditions should lead you to the design of a program and marketing strategy that has the greatest probability of success.

Product

The specific set of services you propose should arise out of the combination of your analysis of what the community is most interested in using and what you are best able to provide. Either individuals' existing awareness of and perceived need for a service, or your confidence that their awareness and perception can be altered, should form the basis for services decisions. This does not preclude professionals from prescribing services in addition to what patients think they need. It does recognize, however, that if patients don't think they need any services at all, they won't contact the professional. Moreover, if they disagree with what the professional thinks they need, they may drop the program or, at a minimum, fail to follow advice.

Place

The location for the program has been discussed. Other "place" issues, however, include hours and days of operation, coverage arrangements for after hours, and appointment and referral arrangements. These also should arise out of a mixture of provider and consumer preference. Consumers may prefer evening hours, or walk-in visits rather than appointments. Providers probably would prefer daytime hours and appointments designed to avoid downtime. Since both ultimately must be satisfied, compromises will be necessary.

Evening hours on some days of the week should be considered. Both market research and trial-and-error can be used to identify the hours most satisfactory to potential customers. Care must be taken to include potential as well as actual patients in research samples to be sure of achieving optimal responses. When providers are made aware of the preferences of their customers and of potential increases in utilization and income, they should be willing to modify hours accordingly.

Price

The use of primary care, especially of relatively optimal services, is very sensitive to price. The charges set for specific services must take into account, first, the standard or competitive charge for the same or similar (as perceived by patients) services. Next, the extent or absence of coverage by prevailing health insurance programs should be considered. Expensive but noncovered services may be subsidized by services that are covered routinely, assuming the insurance payments are not cost based. Third, the extent to which charges will produce income necessary to cover costs must be considered. None of these considerations should dictate price absolutely, since all are critical to the success of specific services.

Promotion

Ideally, promotion should be limited to informing potential patients of the existence of your program, its services hours, (prices?), and location. There are a number of ways in which the awareness of the general public can be enhanced aside from traditional advertising or public service announcements, however. Signs, well lit (if open at night) or at least large and striking (though tasteful) should be used as a constant cue as well as guide to patients coming your way.

A community advisory board provides a promotion mechanism. Members should be encouraged to talk about your program at every opportunity. Free screening services, well-baby clinics, prenatal education classes, CPR training, and other health-related services can be offered by your program, and, where possible, in your facility to acquaint residents with your existence.

The most important promotional device for any health service, however, clearly is word-of-mouth advertising. Customers may be enticed to visit or use your services the first time through all kinds of public relations or advertising gimmicks. However, it is how they perceive the services they receive that determines whether they return and what kind of message they take to their relatives and friends. The importance of pleasing the customer, as well as providing professionally high quality services, should be stressed continually within the program, among all employees.

There is no single recipe for successful planning and implementation of primary care programs. Because they are health services, it is not enough to say simply: find out what they want and give it to them. The idea of selling the sizzle rather than the steak may be fine in other industries, but health is different. On the other hand, if we cannot discover what people want and gear our programs to that, inserting what we feel they need, our efforts are likely to be in vain.

Marketing requires a yielding of professional sovereignty that many health professionals will find uncomfortable. In an era of increasing consumer awareness, greater distrust of authority, and growing competitiveness in the health field, effective marketing is becoming virtually essential to survival.

Chapter 20

Innovative Service Development

Pacific Hospital is a 200-bed acute care general hospital, operated as a not-for-profit community institution. It is located in a well-established urban area, adjacent to an interstate highway exit, and next to a major shopping center. It is a general though full-service hospital, deriving the vast majority of its patients from the immediate urban area, although a significant portion comes from the nearby suburbs. It has enjoyed stable though only average occupancy and has operated slightly in the black consistently for many years.

One of the long-term nuisances in the hospital's program had been its speech and hearing clinic. While accepted as a necessary part of the hospital's overall program, given its emphasis on rehabilitation services, it had been a consistent money loser, despite the internal referrals of stroke and aphasic patients. The speech and hearing clinic was developed as an intrinsic, needed adjunct to the rehabilitation program without any market analysis as to the potential demand for its services.

The volume of patients using the clinic never had been more than a handful, ranging from ten to 15 a week, not enough to justify a full-time staff. Necessary personnel, including trainees from the nearby university programs in audiology and speech therapy, were employed on a part-time basis. While insurance support was available for most patients, the high fixed costs of the clinic, borne by a few, made it impossible for the facility to cover its cost of operation. By 1975, it was losing an average of $3,000 a month and the hospital was sorely pressed to make up such losses anywhere else.

In 1975, the hospital hired a new administrator who rapidly identified the speech and hearing clinic as a major problem area. While the obvious choice seemed to be termination of the program, because of the low volume of internal referrals and few if any outside referrals, the administrator gave the matter careful thought. He brought in a group of audiologists and speech pathologists from around the community to help put the problem in perspective. They insisted that there were large numbers of individuals in the community who *needed* the kinds of services offered by the clinic. The difficulty was in translating that need into effective demand.

One of the local professionals who participated in these discussions expressed a willingness to follow up those convictions with action by taking over the running of the clinic. The administrator set a requirement that the speech and hearing program would have to be self-sustaining within one year, but gave Dr. A, a Ph.D. audiologist, essentially free reign in determining how best to accomplish this objective. While the administrator was less than optimistic, he felt giving Dr. A a chance was a worthwhile gamble, if only to give the hospital a year to phase out its unsuccessful program.

CAPABILITY ANALYSIS

Rather than start with an analysis of the market, Dr. A chose to examine critically the existing scope and capacity of the clinic. Compared to the comprehensive program he had in mind, the current facility and staff were inadequate. He located a large space in one of the other hospital buildings, adequate for his initial purposes and with plenty of room for later expansion. The new space actually was farther from the rehabilitation unit but much more accessible to the public than the former location.

The staff inadequacies were addressed by adding new personnel and replacing part-timers who didn't fit into the kind of program Dr. A had in mind. This caused some ill feelings among staff members who lost their jobs and among other hospital employees as well. Some of the hospital physicians objected to the high-handed way Dr. A was dealing with professional staff, including some of their favorites among older employees.

MARKET ANALYSIS

Dr. A recognized intuitively that the internal inpatient market was totally inadequate as a basis for maintaining a successful clinic. He also could see that the range of services formerly provided in the clinic was inadequate even to the total needs of inpatients, much less the larger speech-and-hearing-impaired community outside the hospital. The clinic had done no previous analysis as to the numbers of potential patients, so no data were available for systematic analysis.

The competition for the market Dr. A had in mind could be divided into three groups. First were other speech and hearing clinics, including one at the university. None actively were seeking patients but were relying on medical referrals from ear, nose, and throat (ENT) specialists in the area. Second were the ENT specialists themselves. These primarily dealt with persons whose hearing or speech difficulties were subject to surgical correction, a small portion of the total market. Third were the hearing aid centers in the area, the most numerous and ubiquitous of the three, though limited to a single, expensive intervention in hearing problems.

An intuitive estimate of the market suggested that the greatest number of persons requiring speech and hearing services were elderly, although adults, school age, and very young children were segments as well. The elderly were likely to be covered by Medicare and/or Medicaid, so financing clinic services should be possible. Other populations could be targeted for development later, once a successful program for the aged was proved.

The competition was anything but frightening. The nongrowth, passive posture of other clinics represented no threat to the untapped market in which Dr. A was interested. ENT specialists tended to focus more on younger people and supplied only surgical remedies. Hearing aid dealers actually were outside the medical system. Individuals usually were not referred by a physician but chose to go to a dealer themselves. The ability of such dealers to test and diagnose hearing problems adequately and determine who should be using what kind of hearing aid certainly was open to question. Moreover, their high prices, which must be paid by the patient in most cases, left them vulnerable.

In designing his program, Dr. A decided he would emphasize a comprehensive, one-stop service clinic at which all speech and hearing problems could be diagnosed accurately and a full range of therapeutic options offered. Where nonsurgical therapy was required, the clinic would provide it. When surgery was indicated, the clinic would refer patients to ENT specialists on the hospital's medical staff. Should a hearing aid be indicated, the clinic would provide it.

This latter decision was controversial. It long had been a principle of the American Speech and Hearing Association (ASHA) that its members would not indulge in the highly profitable competitive and somewhat unsavory business of hearing aid sales. This overt dealing with a product, one available over the counter in countless centers and stores around the country, didn't seem appropriate for health professionals. Moreover, the traditionally high markup (up to 300 percent over cost) would leave the health professionals open to charges of price gouging.

Dr. A saw the situation from a different light. Clearly, individuals with hearing problems should have access to the best, most comprehensive set of services available rather than take a chance on the one-solution products of hearing aid dealers. Moreover, if the price of hearing aids was such a deterrent, the clinic would offer them at cost. Because it was a health care organization, part of a hospital, the clinic found that in most cases Medicare and Medicaid would cover the cost of hearing aids provided in the clinic as prosthetic devices. This further added to the list of advantages offered by the clinic.

Arrangements were made with hearing aid manufacturers so that the clinic could offer a number of brands, rather than the single-brand options usually available at hearing aid dealers. Commitments to discounts were arranged based on the volume of visits expected. A physician was recruited to provide medical supervision and backup for the clinic. A new staff was hired and trained for this comprehensive approach to speech and hearing care. The full array of interventions for speech and hearing problems would be available through a single clinic, serving the entire metropolitan area.

PROMOTION

The director of the program, Dr. A, was at his best in the promotional side of marketing, although he had some unwitting assistance. He first planned a news conference to announce the opening of the clinic and, thanks to the controversial nature of the program, was able to attract substantial coverage. The administration and medical staff of the hospital were less than delighted with this publicity, especially since they had not been informed of the conference in advance. However, it generated much attention to and awareness of the clinic and its new program.

At the news conference, the director cited the lack of comprehensive, continuous services for the speech/hearing impaired, made some remarks critical of hearing aid dealers, and presented the clinic's response to the community. He announced that free screening services would be available and that hearing aids would be sold at cost. This news was given front-page coverage, perhaps in accurate anticipation of the controversy that would arise.

The local hearing aid dealers' association became involved and sued the hospital, complaining of defamation and restraint of trade. This suit kept the clinic in the news for quite some time after opening. The publicity aroused much interest in the market and was followed by an average of 125 appointment requests a day. Within a week of opening, the clinic's appointment times were booked three months in advance.

As the program developed, further promotional efforts were undertaken. The free screening program was taken out to the community to nursing homes and senior citizens' centers. A mobile van provided free screening at shopping malls, churches, fairs, and industries. Staff members, once only two in number but grown to 26, spoke to interested social clubs and luncheon groups. Pamphlets describing the clinic's program were distributed at public gatherings. Physicians' offices had pamphlets available for their patients.

Messages describing the clinic, or one of its screening programs, were carried regularly in the media as public service announcements.

Past patients were remembered. Christmas and birthday cards were sent to patients, plays using sign language were presented for deaf children, and a Santa Claus who could use sign language was available at each year's Christmas party. Patients returned periodically to the clinic for follow-up visits and retesting and were made to feel like members of its large family.

Additional promotional outreach efforts were instituted. Free hearing tests were administered to all newborn babies in the hospital. Children born in the hospital were invited to have a preschool hearing evaluation. Parents were encouraged to bring in their children to identify speech and hearing problems early, before they showed up as school difficulties. Children with learning disabilities often were identified and special diagnostic and therapy programs were developed for them as well.

The hospital's clinic became a regional speech and hearing program for the entire metropolitan area and even beyond. It diagnosed and treated or referred virtually all speech and hearing problems that afflict individuals. It succeeded beyond the requirements and wildest dreams of the administrator, and is still growing. It serves as an example for innovating hospitals as to how widely they might look in identifying and responding to health markets.

MARKETING ANALYSIS

The first lesson that can be learned from this case is an important maxim, usually expressed as:

no amount of planning is a substitute for good dumb luck!

Put another way, it does not always take systematic market analysis and development for a program to succeed if the climate's right. This case was chosen consciously for inclusion here as a demonstration of the fact that intuitive marketing decision making will work, provided the situation is ripe for it. Hosts of successful programs have developed before people could spell marketing, much less apply it "properly." Similarly, some of the most expensive marketing minds in the country created the Edsel.

ENVIRONMENT AND COMPETITION

The major advantage this hospital enjoyed in developing its speech and hearing clinic had to do with its competition. First, the nature of the competition tended to prevent it from opposing the clinic's development or from being able to retain its own markets once the clinic was under way. Other speech and hearing clinics basically were passive, waiting for enough referrals from physicians to keep busy but not actively seeking new markets. Physicians specializing in ENT were well-established competitors, but only for that small portion of the market where surgical solutions to their problems were appropriate. Hearing aid dealers were out of the mainstream of medical care, mostly limited to one brand of hearing aids that represented one solution to hearing problems, and unable to compete on price. The ability of the clinic to sell hearing aids at cost, and to get even those costs picked up by Medicare/Medicaid, represented an enormous price advantage.

Such circumstances are rare in the health care field, though by no means unique. It could be argued that with such a favorable competitive environment, the clinic would have succeeded without effort. As a rule, however, it should not be assumed that the approach this clinic used should be followed for all new program developments, or even by other health care organizations that decide to develop speech and hearing services. For example, being sued may be good publicity, but losing the suit could represent some hardship. Disparaging the competition can have negative repercussions, especially in the health field. Failing to clear news conferences with others in the organization could be fatal in some circumstances.

Dr. A at least intuitively recognized the strengths of his proposed program relative to the competition. He perhaps missed some opportunities to *use* his competitors as possible referral sources, however, by running roughshod over them. Moreover, the marginal medical identity of his program protected it from the kinds of ethics of advertising concerns likely to emerge in a strictly traditional health care program requiring services by M.D.s as well as Ph.D.s. In a sense, of course, the opposition his clinic aroused outside the hospital helped give him the publicity he wanted. It tended at first to sensitize the medical community against the clinic, however, as a rowdy, somewhat unsavory program.

MARKETS

The market segment identification by Dr. A, again determined intuitively rather than systematically, was particularly astute. By determining accurately which were the major markets (aged, preschool and newborn children), he recognized immediately that the then existing program was off target. The ability to shift a program completely away from its present market toward a new one is rare among health programs. The combination of a money-losing history, a new administrator, and the new director, especially given the carte blanche power conferred on him as long as the financial crisis could be overcome, made this a unique rather than a common opportunity.

STRATEGY

Dr. A approached these markets through an effective combination of product, price, and place. By developing a comprehensive rather than a narrow service program, he offered one-stop convenience and could promise a response tailored to the needs of each patient. The connection with the hospital and ready referrals for medical care enhanced the confidence individuals placed in clinic services and extended even to the nontraditional hearing aid business. By taking screening services to fairs, shopping centers, nursing homes, senior citizen centers, and nurseries, the clinic's offerings were made maximally accessible to the markets Dr. A was trying to reach. The price advantages he could offer by selling hearing aids at cost and getting Medicare/Medicaid coverage for them, was unique and overwhelming good fortune.

The clinic's promotional efforts took advantage of the interest of the news media in conflict and in dramatic innovations. Not all new programs can expect to receive such favorable or extensive attention, however. The fact that the hearing aid dealers helped inadvertently in this promotional effort can't be counted on in other circumstances. The offering of a unique program to a large community has enabled the clinic to take advantage of public service announcement activities by the media. The clinic's not quite medical nature has freed it from normal medical constraints on advertising. All these advantages are unlikely to be repeated, even if the same hospital develops additional programs.

No projection ever was made of potential demand for the clinic's services. The program grew like Topsy, adding staff and equipment in response to demand more often than in anticipation of it. No systematic market analysis was made of the major market—the aged—as to how many potentially needed, would be interested in, or could pay for the clinic's services. Dr. A was fortunate in finding space with plenty of room for expansion and in being in a major metropolitan area with ready access to the personnel necessary to offer and augment clinic services. The intuitive estimates of Dr. A and his colleagues were indeed correct, but not recommended for all programs. In most circumstances, a more deliberate estimate of demand and concomitant development of service capacity is advised.

The clinic achieved a resounding success relative to the patient market, but has not done as well among physicians. It does not receive as many referrals as it might, in part because of the notoriety created by the lawsuit and in part because of its nonmedical director. The administration of the hospital was not kept informed about, nor consulted, regarding the clinic's plans, and has not as favorable an attitude regarding the clinic or Dr. A as it might have. It is likely that much more careful supervision will attend any future program developments by Dr. A, although the success of the program gives him a strong "track record" credibility.

The typical health care approach to marketing was followed only in part by Dr. A, much to his credit. Rather than limit his thinking to what his profession or other speech and hearing clinics normally do, he recognized the potentially wider need and demand in the community. He recognized the distinct limitations of mobility common to his intended markets and took his services at least in part to them rather than waiting for them to come to him.

The development of the clinic followed a logical if reactive sequence, beginning with the largest market where the clinic had the greatest advantages—the aged. As it expanded its scope to include children, however, it began to encounter fewer market advantages and stiffer competition from medical practitioners. Hearing aids no longer were the product sold, but treatment and counseling, and results tended to be less dramatic than where surgery was possible. Both the clinic and ENT specialists share the advantages of being able to seek reimbursement through health insurance.

Dr. A is certainly the kind of personal dynamo who can design, develop, and implement a program without much assistance and even in the face of opposition. On the other hand, his cavalier relations with administration and medical staff have left ill feelings that could have been avoided. Perhaps the two inevitably occur together, but a systematic market analysis might have saved him some strained relationships. Of course, it could always be the case that waiting for a systematic market analysis could have resulted in the clinic's missing the boat if another innovative dynamo had decided on a similar program and forged ahead based on intuition.

A success, especially one as overwhelming as this speech and hearing clinic, is always a difficult phenomenon to criticize. Indeed, it may be partly sour grapes to suggest that Dr. A did everything or anything wrong when things turned out so well. Much of what systematic market analysis would have revealed was estimated intuitively yet correctly by the director. On the other hand, there is always a danger that we will accept such successes uncritically and believe the process followed must be correct if it worked. Failures, fortunately, are more likely to be examined, and better lessons learned.

DISCUSSION QUESTIONS

1. Are there market segments (such as the aged) for which you could develop a new service program (e.g., day care, nutrition services, speech and hearing)?
2. Do you now have the basic capability of providing those services or would you have to start from scratch?
3. What is your present competition and what does it offer in terms of product, price, and place to that segment?
4. What other organizations have a better basic capacity to provide such services (personnel, equipment, facilities, location) and might decide to do so?
5. What can you do that is better than existing and potential competition?
6. What would be the impact on your organization if you succeeded in implementing such a program? At what levels of utilization?
7. What internal groups must be won over to the idea for it to succeed?
8. What external groups?
9. How might the program be developed so as to improve the probability that internal groups will support it?
10. Can you involve potential consumers or referral agencies in developing the program?
11. What groups or individuals might oppose the development and for what reasons?
12. Can they be won over or is it necessary to defeat them?
13. What strategies can you use for either?
14. What benefits can you promise to interested groups as a result of implementing the program and at what costs?
15. How can you communicate most effectively to the precise segments of the market most likely to use the program?
16. What message will be most likely to stir their interest?

Chapter 21

Developmental Opportunities

To a great extent, the "need" and potential demand for health services is virtually infinite. As inpatient and conventional medical services programs become increasingly constrained by government regulation and reimbursement, and increasingly competitive, interest inevitably will grow in opportunities for diversification. Growth is accepted as an almost universal measure of success, and in many areas, growth will be possible only through development of new programs.

Great care should be taken in examining new program alternatives. It is a common phenomenon for almost any development, even before it is tried and proved, to spawn competitors. Unless a new program can be expected to succeed against potential competition, it probably should not be attempted. Clear identification of success measures, expectations, and the actions in the market necessary to achieve success should be spelled out and analyzed relative to each opportunity.

Many development opportunities are related closely and should be considered together. If each is supportive of the other, promoting greater and more efficient use of facilities, equipment, and personnel, it may be advantageous to develop them together, even though the initial investment may be larger. Multiple development of interacting options may provide multiple avenues for success, enabling generally positive outcomes, even if parts of the program fall short.

Virtually all new program opportunities require conscious marketing analysis and effort, in contrast to more traditional programs dependent on the successful recruitment of physicians. Most can be developed with relatively little capital investment through use of existing facilities or leasing of space. All entail some risk, however, since marketing and resources development costs are likely to be significant. Most have some promise of developing additional users of traditional services through disease detection or referral.

All these programs are susceptible to conventional though adapted marketing techniques and all require some formal approach to promotion (advertising or publicity). All are subject to some internal resistance or at least concern because they both extend the bounds of traditional medical services and border on the corporate practice of health care. All may have to be "sold" to support publics as well as potential users of specific services, both through design (product, price, place) and persuasion (promotion).

The following sample of developmental opportunities represents programs that have been developed successfully in at least a few settings. Each of the ten opportunities is sketched only briefly, with emphasis on the marketing implications of each. Those interested in pursuing any particular program opportunity further are advised to check the professional literature to identify who has experience with each, as well as to gain further insight into the particulars of each.

BEHAVIOR MODIFICATION PROGRAMS

The general area of behavior modification programs covers a host of specific services. These include diet and nutrition programs, stop-smoking clinics, exercise promotion, phobia clinics, etc. They generally are fairly remote from traditional medical care and, in any community, are likely to be offered by a number of diverse organizations. Most include some sort of consciousness-raising together with group support and educational approaches to modifying undesirable behavior.

Individuals may enter such programs on referral from physicians and social service agencies, or on their own. Industries may encourage workers or executives to partake of specific services, such as exercise or diet clinics. Many persons are likely to be interested potentially in more than one program. The health care organization has some advantages in providing such services where linkage to medical care is useful. Medical testing and monitoring is helpful for exercise programs and diet clinics. Psychiatric backup services may be worthwhile for any behavior modification program where severe emotional problems are involved.

Health care organizations are likely to enjoy credibility advantages over unfamiliar single-purpose agencies. They also may be able to use existing facilities such as physical therapy areas for exercise. Care must be taken in assigning facility costs and overhead to such programs, lest the costs push charges above competitive levels.

The critical market factors in achieving success in such programs are likely to be place and promotion. Evening hours and local sites are likely to be essential in attracting working people to regular meetings. Schools and churches may be available as inexpensive facilities, and both are likely to have accessible parking. Price can be adjusted based on the competition and the size of groups attracted to the programs. Dieticians, physical therapists, psychologists, social workers, and other professionals already working in health organizations may be interested in staffing the programs for extra income.

Promotion of such services can be carried out formally via public service announcements or advertising. Word-of-mouth communication is likely to be most effective. Successful clients of such programs may be employed as outreach workers on a part-time basis. Their enthusiastic descriptions of what the programs did for them are likely to be very persuasive, especially to friends and acquaintances in their own communities.

Since the capital outlay for these programs is very low, all provide opportunities for toe-in-the-water approaches. Some preliminary market research as to the level of interest, attitudes toward the potential sponsoring organization, and nature of the competition still would be worthwhile, however. Where use of ancillary services is promoted (lab tests in diet programs, stress tests and EKGs for exercise services, etc.), additional revenue should be anticipated.

While behavior modification programs are likely to begin with specific focuses, they may include attention to the general area of how to use health services. Efforts may be made to cover self-care, describing what average informed persons can do for themselves and when they should see a health professional. Such programs may even include a product, such as a home care kit, including thermometer, blood pressure device, and charts and booklets describing how to deal with specific problems. There is likely to be professional resistance to the promotion of self-care, but such programs can be targeted at eliminating or demarketing inappropriate use of services, such as emergency rooms for routine problems. A telephone advisory service should be made available in conjunction with a program to answer questions not covered in the kit.

The expected impact of such a program on the use of the organization's existing services should be addressed specifically.

BIRTHING CENTERS

There is a growing interest in alternative approaches to obstetrics. The high-cost sterile institutional experience of hospital obstetric programs is being questioned increasingly. One source of objection appears to be related to feminist resistance to turning over control to predominantly male obstetricians. Another is the expensive, impersonal environment. A third comes from the feeling that birth is a natural phenomenon and ought to take place in a natural setting.

The result of these attitudes is the growth of home deliveries and freestanding birth centers. Yet, from a medical perspective, many of the clients of such alternatives are taking a dreadful risk. Primiparous mothers always are question marks with regard to pelvic size, for example, and the potential for serious delivery problems may not be apparent in many cases until too late. If the lack of quick medical response produces damaged babies and mothers, the cost and personal advantages of these alternatives may not be worth the risk.

Hospitals may be able to offer the advantages of the alternatives without the disadvantages. Birthing centers may be developed adjacent to or even as part of the hospital. Given the low utilization of obstetric services, hospitals may be able to offer both the traditional medical and the newer alternative approaches to obstetrics. The alternative program with its lower cost and homelike atmosphere may be used up to the point that medical intervention is deemed necessary.

As the number of births per mother decreases, and because of the higher risk of the first birth, the major market for promoting an alternative birthing center program would be the primiparous mother. Prenatal education classes can be offered by or in the hospital, with an opportunity to visit the birthing center included. Obstetricians and family practitioners on the medical staff will have to be approached carefully in order to gain their support of and participation in such a program.

For the community, the advantages of a hospital-based birthing center over traditional obstetrics lie in the lower cost and potentially higher acceptability by mothers. In contrast to home birth or even nonhospital birthing centers, there may be advantages of lower maternal and infant mortality and morbidity and the opportunity for a quicker response during unexpected critical periods that occur during the birth process.

For physicians, while loss of income is likely compared to home or other nonphysician-attended birth, the hospital-based alternative gives them the assurance that medical assistance will be available on a standby basis. The hospital gains added use of existing facilities, although it will lose revenue compared to traditional obstetrics since the charge per day, delivery charge, and length of stay will be significantly lower.

GERIATRIC PROGRAMS

Geriatrics includes a host of program development opportunities—day-care programs, home health services, traditional long-term care, weekend or episodic custodial services, homemaker services, and ambulatory programs geared to the particular needs of elderly populations. If a complementary set of such services can be offered, the advantages of a one-site, one-sponsor program can be substantial. Potential recipients of such services are likely to move from need of one type to need of another and back, as well as benefit from inpatient and traditional outpatient medical services on occasion.

Since the number of elderly persons in the population is growing faster than the population as a whole, and since the number of superelderly (over 75, over 85) is rising fastest of all, the market for such services is bound to expand. Moreover, as interest in containing health care costs intensifies, support for alternatives to institutional services is bound to grow.

The advantages of close medical monitoring in a program of comprehensive geriatric services are particularly strong. The elderly are likely to suffer from a number of at least partially disabling conditions, including hypertension, hearing problems, nutritional difficulties, neurological and circulatory problems, and pharmaceutical conflicts. Having medical supervision readily available should promote more effective detection of and response to such problems. Having a whole range of alternative services available should prevent the overuse of unnecessarily expensive ones or delayed use of appropriate care.

A full range of related services also offers cost advantages. Dietary programs housed in institutions can serve as sources of meals-on-wheels, day care, or nutritional services. Inpatient physical and occupational therapy facilities can be used for outpatient care and exercise programs. The advantages of increased volumes should offer economies of scale in most cases.

Moreover, the availability of easy medical standby services seems to be of great concern to elderly persons and their families. This availability should be stressed in promotional efforts, although word-of-mouth advertising is equally important. Referrals from social service agencies should be encouraged. Churches and senior citizen centers represent logical places for permanent displays.

The chief disadvantage in geriatric programs is the financial risk. Generally, while elderly populations need more services, they have less income to pay for them. Their health insurance is likely to be limited in coverage of anything but traditional inpatient care. Unless and until the cost advantages of alternative programs are demonstrated to government, the financial risk of geriatric programs is likely to remain high.

HOSPICE

The idea of programs offering comprehensive medical, psychological, and social services to the terminally ill and their families through hospices is receiving growing support. The traditional hospital treatment of the dying has been found to be as lacking as that of the newborn, for many of the same reasons. As concern grows over death with dignity, and as the extremely high cost of heroic efforts to maintain minimal quality of life is recognized, interest in hospice programs is bound to grow. Moreover, as the population shifts toward more aged, and as chronic disease grows concomitantly, the demand for hospice services is likely to be increasing also.

Whether an organization should develop a hospice program is a function of its own capabilities and commitment as well as potential demand. Making long-term commitments to serving the needs of the terminally ill and their families requires special attitudes as well as services. Most physicians and other health professionals view death as failure and are uncomfortable with the idea of providing a supportive atmosphere to accommodate the end of life. Regular confrontation with death can have a severe psychological impact on those who work in a hospice program.

A hospice requires a rather full set of related services: inpatient, outpatient, and home care, for both dying patient and the family. Whether such services fit well with existing programs should be examined carefully along with the willingness and ability to handle the psychological and emotional conse-quences. Institutions that traditionally have emphasized high-technology medical interventions are less appropriate than those that have focused on personal care and emotional support.

As with geriatric services, there may be significant financial risk in a hos-pice program. Health insurance may well cover the inpatient and medical portions of a hospice program but neglect the psychosocial and home serv-ices. Persons dying of chronic diseases may well have exhausted their insur-ance, and personal and even family finances before reaching the point of needing hospice services.

Successful development of a hospice program requires the creation and maintenance of strong referral linkages with social agencies and other health organizations. Both promotional communication and regular feedback on specific patients to physicians and agencies that refer them to the hospice should be conducted carefully. Here, too, word-of-mouth communication from families served by a hospice program is likely to have the greatest credibility and impact.

HOTEL SERVICES

Major specialty service institutions are likely to encounter numerous situa-tions in which a demand for nonmedical accommodations is generated by a medical care program. Patients coming from out of town for a series of outpatient tests often will have to stay at least overnight, perhaps for a num-ber of days. The Mayo Clinic in Rochester, Minnesota, keeps a host of hotels in business. Families of patients coming from some distance for surgery on an outpatient or inpatient basis will need accommodations nearby. Patients and families coming for a series of therapeutic services, such as radiation therapy or a chemotherapeutic series, also will want a place to stay. Individuals on home dialysis, or other chronic disease patients requiring intensive periodic checkups, may need regular accommodations.

Hotels, in many situations, are either not located conveniently or simply not well suited to the particular need of such persons. In many circumstances, hospitals or large medical groups may find it both appropriate and rewarding to develop their own hotel services geared to the unusual circumstances of patients and their families. Old hospital buildings, or even unused portions of relatively modern facilities, may be converted to such use.

The use of facilities immediately adjacent to or part of the hospital offers unique advantages in terms of ready access to the institution in the event of an emergency. The very proximity of the hospital's resources will be reassuring even when they are not needed. Patients, families, and other visitors housed in such accommodations may be fed through the hospital's dietary service, providing additional revenue.

Hotel programs also may be used to accommodate physicians attending continuing education programs, potential physician recruits and their families, other potential employees coming for interviews, etc. If the volume of guests of some types proves insufficient to generate adequate occupancy, many other types are likely to be available.

Opposition to such programs can be counted on from existing hotel and motel operators, and certificate-of-need approval probably is necessary. There is high risk in any large capital investment such as this, so careful research as to the potential demand, willingness to use the service proposed, and price sensitivity is recommended strongly. Patient origin studies and surveys of current patients and families arriving from significant distances should be carried out. Institutions proposing such developments should be sure that significant advantages will be expected and received by people using their hotel services as compared to competitive offerings.

INDUSTRIAL HEALTH

The general area of industrial health can include a number of specific services. At the simplest level, new employees may be given preemployment or insurance physicals, for example. Expanding further, employees in risky industries may be monitored regularly for conditions affecting their lungs, blood, etc. The working environment itself may be monitored for hazards, either of accidental injury or occupational disease, including stress from noise, employment pressure, or other occupational causes.

Marketing services to industry is a slightly different problem from marketing directly to the public. First, the advantages to the specific industry of having a health service program must be identified and designed into the program. Second, the advantages of your organization as the source of the program must be clear and real. The advantages of marketing to industry lie in the large number of patients who come with each industrial concern recruited, in contrast to direct marketing to the general public. Similarly, the large volume of use that can result should enable the organization to offer high quality services at reasonable costs.

Environmental surveillance and corrective programs have to be coordinated closely with prevailing Occupational Safety and Health Act (OSHA) regulations and programs. Since these are preventive services, they will not produce referrals for related care. Routine physicals or employee screening programs, however, will identify persons needing follow-up medical care. Such referrals should be handled carefully to avoid angering the local medical society or the institution's own medical staff. The ability and willingness of the organization to handle both screening and referrals should be clearly present or carefully developed before such a program is undertaken.

Depending on relative location and the size of the population served, screening and routine physical exams may be offered at the industrial site rather than in the organization's own facility. Prices must be set so as to compete not only with other organizations that do or might offer similar services but with the industrial client's own capacity to provide the service.

Promotion of such programs to industry almost has to be carried out by direct contact. Initial approaches may be made on a one-to-one basis to nearby industrial sites, while more general approaches can be made through speaking at gatherings of business persons (e.g., Rotary or Chamber of Commerce luncheons). Large industries are a logical first step for development, although once the program is developed, smaller business establishments may be recruited also

OUTPATIENT SURGERY

Outpatient surgery is an already well-established alternative to traditional patterns of care. Whether freestanding or hospital-based, such programs offer distinct cost, convenience, and quality advantages. By saving an overnight stay in the hospital, recipients enjoy reduced charges and less disruption of their lives, though the former advantage may be eliminated by the vagaries of health insurance. The psychological and social advantages of outpatient surgery are considerable, as the risk tends to be perceived as very small when surgery can be done without an overnight stay.

The biggest consideration in developing an outpatient surgery program probably should be whether it represents simply an alternative approach to providing the same services to the same markets or is likely to involve new services or new markets. If a hospital's inpatient surgery program is keeping many beds full, and use of operating room facilities is optimal, switching a large number of individuals to outpatient status simply will decrease inpatient revenues and lower occupancy. If an outpatient program produces greater use of operating room facilities in a hospital where lack of beds reduced surgical workloads, or enables an organization to see more patients, the benefits are likely to be greater.

At least three markets are critical to a successful outpatient surgery program. First and foremost are surgeons and referring physicians who must accept outpatient surgery as superior or at least equal to the inpatient alternative in terms of their values: safety for the patient, income for the physician, malpractice risk, acceptability to the family, etc. Second are the patients and families themselves, who may resist or welcome an outpatient alternative, depending on how they see themselves affected. Third are the health insurance companies whose coverage policies may discriminate inadvertently against outpatient surgery.

All three are interrelated closely, since the judgments by decisionmakers (referring physician, surgeon, patient/family) all will be affected by cost and quality perceptions.

The hospital-based program probably offers the best backup in the event of unforeseen difficulties, though careful selection of patients enables freestanding programs to do well also. Whether hospital or medical group sponsorship provides a marketing advantage can be determined only by surveying the potential market (physicians and patients) regarding reputation. In many situations, offering outpatient surgery is becoming virtually a necessity in providing comprehensive services and demonstrating cost containment to regulatory agencies.

PRIMARY MEDICAL CARE

Specialty hospitals and medical groups increasingly are confronting similar disturbing realities. Previous sources of referrals slowly but inexorably are drying up. Smaller communities and hospitals increasingly are developing their own specialized services, except for the most sophisticated. As family practitioners and general internists replace general practitioners, the new physicians are less likely to refer patients to other physicians for routine surgery, medical care, or obstetrics. Institutions and organizations that have relied on referrals from outside their control have seen diminished utilization and revenue.

For such organizations, the development of their own primary care programs offers two distinct advantages. First, it promotes greater use of facilities and equipment as individuals increase their use of services. Second, it creates new, internal sources of referrals for specialized services. The proximity of specialists, relationships with colleagues that develop, and mutual economic advantages tend to firm up referral patterns when the organization sponsors its own primary care programs.

These are likely to be barriers, however. Specialist groups and hospitals may resent the loss of power that comes from bringing in a number of primary practitioners. Unless the specialists yield a little on privileges related to simple surgery and obstetrics, they may be unable to attract new primary care physicians. If they do yield, they may be going counter to their own principles and automatically be decreasing the percentage of cases that will be referred. They may see the introduction of primary care services as a dilution of their specialist image, as well.

Sponsorship of primary care programs is likely to be somewhat riskier for hospitals than for medical groups. If physicians are recruited for the primary care program on the basis of salary compensation or contract, they eventually may become disenchanted with the constraints of the institutional linkage and strike out on their own. This could leave the institution holding the bag of a primary care facility without patients. A medical group, in contrast, can make the primary care practitioner a full and equal participant in the group's affairs and income, making retention more likely.

Populations in truly isolated rural regions, or areas where residence turnover is high, are better prospects for new primary care programs. Care must be taken to be sure that persons in such areas are willing to change their way of dealing with primary care needs and have sufficient numbers and income to support such a program financially. The reason for any current absence of primary care physicians should be examined carefully. Perhaps these reasons will represent a problem that a sponsored program can solve, or an insurmountable barrier to successful development by anyone.

SCREENING SERVICES

Screening programs are aimed at early detection of chronic conditions that can be corrected or at least controlled through medical care, diet, etc. Effective screening programs are being carried out for diabetes, hypertension, glaucoma, blood cholesterol/triglycerides, visual, hearing, and other common but frequently undetected problems. The benefit to the community is substantial: early detection of major health threats, potential reduction in costs if early treatment prevents acute levels of need, and identification of major communitywide problems that might be dealt with preventively (e.g., lung diseases resulting from occupational or environmental pollution).

The key to screening programs is to make the product as simple as possible, a service that can be done quickly, without pain or embarrassment, yet is accurate. Moreover, screening should be done only for conditions where early intervention significantly improves the quality of results, or at least reduces the cost of care. Screening that merely promises early identification without changing the consequences is more harmful than beneficial.

Place considerations suggest locating screening services as convenient as possible to where large numbers of persons congregate: downtown parks or malls, shopping centers, etc. Such services also may be offered at the institution if a second purpose is to raise the level of community awareness of its existence, to impress individuals favorably with a new building, or similar reasons. The price normally should be free, both of out-of-pocket costs and of any discomfort.

Referral of persons with positive findings should be handled very carefully. An aggressive, competitive approach would be to refer everyone possible to the organization's own treatment programs or medical staff. Except in a one-hospital or one-clinic community, however, it may be better to refer them to their own physician if they have one, and offer the organization as a choice only to those who claim no personal physician relationship. Most persons probably will choose the organization as the source of follow-up care voluntarily. Referrals to the organization's own medical staff should be made according to arrangements agreed upon by that staff to avoid internal squabbling.

Promotion of screening services can be carried out legitimately through public service announcements in the news media. Schools and social service agencies often will be willing to promote screening services through announcements and posters. National organizations such as heart associations and cancer societies will be able to supply materials and assistance. Joint sponsorship with such organizations may be necessary as a *quid pro quo,* but should be well worth the price. The specific benefits to the organization of new patient referrals as well as general public relations advantages makes screening for problems the institution is prepared to handle a typically rewarding option.

SPORTS MEDICINE

With increasing interest in exercise, and perhaps the likelihood that we'll all be doing more walking, running, and biking as gasoline supplies dry up, there are bound to be increasing numbers of sore muscles, joints, feet, knees, etc. As a result, there will be a growing market for sports medicine programs. Most of us can't afford a full-time trainer but can benefit from occasional advice, diagnosis, and treatment of the kinds of aches, pains, strains, sprains, muscle and joint problems common to athletes.

Sports medicine programs are likely to appeal to any area of the country where casual involvement in sports or athletic activity is common. Joggers, bikers, hikers, tennis and racquetball players, playground basketball enthusiasts, and softball players are subject to frequent and even chronic problems. While a physician's services are necessary on occasion, a physical therapist will be very useful in initiating and monitoring corrective exercise programs, hydrotherapy, flexibility conditioning, and other direct services.

Consultations by orthopedists, podiatrists, and physical medicine and rehabilitation specialists may be called for on occasion. The equipment required for a sports medicine program need not be extensive or expensive, although considerable space is needed to carry on diagnostic therapy and exercise activities on a regular basis. Hours will have to be tailored to the market segments targeted, with much activity expected on Mondays for the weekend superstars. Close links should be established with exercise promotion and monitoring programs.

The newsworthy event approach to publicity is a logical choice for sports medicine programs. If local sports heroes can be encouraged to visit, test out the facilities, etc., the "legitimacy" of the program may be established. Descriptions of services and hours should be placed in areas frequented by sports participants—Y's, community centers, tennis and racquetball clubs, and jogging areas. As with most health service programs, however, the comments of satisfied customers provide the most credible and effective advertising.

Index

About the Author

ROBIN E. SCOTT MACSTRAVIC teaches health planning, marketing, and program development in the Graduate Program in Health Services Administration and Planning at the University of Washington in Seattle. Prior to his current faculty appointment, he taught similar subjects at the Medical College of Virginia in Richmond. He began his health career in the marketing division of Michigan Blue Cross and has held positions in hospital administration and health planning. He has consulted with over 20 hospitals on the development of primary medical care programs and the determination of resource requirements. Dr. MacStravic is the author of *Marketing Health Care* and *Determining Health Needs*.